EVOLVING
MEDICINE

EVOLVING MEDICINE

How to Make the Art of Healing Healthy Again

MAGDA MONTASIR

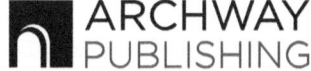

ARCHWAY
PUBLISHING

Archway Publishing books may be ordered through booksellers or by contacting:

Archway Publishing
1663 Liberty Drive
Bloomington, IN 47403
www.archwaypublishing.com
1 (888) 242-5904

Because of the dynamic nature of the Internet, any web addresses or links contained in this book may have changed since publication and may no longer be valid. The views expressed in this work are solely those of the author and do not necessarily reflect the views of the publisher, and the publisher hereby disclaims any responsibility for them.

Any people depicted in stock imagery provided by Thinkstock are models, and such images are being used for illustrative purposes only. Certain stock imagery © Thinkstock.

ISBN: 978-1-4808-1769-2 (sc)
ISBN: 978-1-4808-1770-8 (e)

Library of Congress Control Number: 2015906070

Print information available on the last page.

Archway Publishing rev. date: 4/27/2015

CONTENTS

ACKNOWLEDGMENT

I am deeply grateful to the highly professional diligent coordinator, editors and the rest of the customer support team of, "Archway at Simon and Schuster Publishing Company," for accepting my manuscript and making my book a success.

My appreciation also goes to everybody who granted me the copyright permission to include their illustrations in my book, as they appear in the list, whether they are companies like Bayer, US government departments, or personal owners, two charged me licensing fees, the remainder allowed me to use them for free. Special thanks to "Marcel Zurreck, in Switzerland who was the first to respond and requested to read the book when published and "Yvonne Frost" who sent me one of their books as a courtesy.

First I'd like to thank Maha Issa the tour guide who showed us around in the old country explaining in detail the meaning and history of what we were viewing with awe and delight in the archeological sites.

I would like to credit Margaret Moustapha Ph.D. Professor Emeritus, Cal State University, L.A. who was the first to give me hints for how to self edit the manuscript before presenting it to the publisher. When she is asked what she teaches she answers: I teach teachers how to teach."

Ismail I. Eldumiati, Ph.D. A Bell Labs fellow and a senior executive with broad experience in engineering and corporate management; he pioneered development in microprocessors, digital signal processors and digital video processing leading to advances in digital communications, high definition video standards and managed R&D, design and development organizations in the US and other countries, who assisted in technological details.

And Virginia Ghoniem, Principal, Darby Avenue Elementary school, who with her review was influential in encouraging me to go ahead with the project.

Last but not least my deep appreciation goes to my husband who inspired me and so patiently and lovingly stood behind me. He literarily did while I was using his computer telling me: "do this and don't do that, and exclude this and include that."

And I am indebted to my Granddaughter "Gianna El Bayar." for her beautiful artwork. She is the one who inspired me to write this book when she said; "I can't wait to see how technology will change in the next ten years." She made me wonder how the future of medicine is going to be.

ABOUT THE AUTHOR

The author is a retired medical doctor. She studied, practiced, worked in research projects and taught in USA and abroad. She has a doctoral degree in Tropical Medicine and Infectious Disease, and is Board Certified in Anatomical and Clinical pathology, and was the director of a hospital laboratory. She used to be a member of several medical associations including Tropical Medicine and Hygiene, American medical, Arab American Medical. The only membership she is still keeping is the College of American Pathologists. She published several articles in Egyptian British and American medical journals.

Realizing the difference in the practice of medicine between three generations of physicians in her own family and comparing health care systems in different countries she started to examine the history of healing and found it fascinating to write about and wonder about how its future will be.

She is the anonymous author of "Biography of an unknown"

PREFACE

With the passage of the Affordable Care Act, the American concern regarding health care rose from simmering to exploding into the public sphere. The act, commonly referred to as Obamacare because of Barrack Obama's adamancy to change the health-care system as his legacy, is now the law of the land and here to stay. The Affordable Care Act was passed and signed into law in 2010. It has survived challenge from the Supreme Court and numerous attempts in Congress to repeal or defund it. When the health-care exchange opened, allowing people to enroll, the demand exceeded all expectations. In fact, the sheer volume of people wanting to know more about the different options and to enroll in one of the many choices available overwhelmed the exchanges.

The Affordable Care Act was needed because there were around 40 million uninsured American citizens at the time, amounting to 16 percent of the US population. These people chose not to buy health insurance because they were young and healthy and felt they wouldn't need it, or because they were in working families who could not afford it. When these uninsured individuals got sick or were involved in an accident, they were compelled to go to the emergency room for free care, and taxpayers had to carry the brunt.

Obamacare was also necessary because insurance companies had strict regulations in place to remain in the black. They denied coverage or treatment of preexisting conditions, or they charged higher premiums in such situations. Many times, insurance companies dropped or restricted benefits when the customer consumed a lot of resources or cost them more than expected. They also charged more for females in their childbearing period of life.

The preceding regulations and the growing unaffordability of health care led toward the need to reform the system. The reforms included mandates including the following: an employer mandate, where large employers and small businesses with twenty-five or more full-time workers had to cover those employees. The individual mandate required everybody to carry adequate coverage, and young adults can be covered by their parents' insurance carrier until the age of twenty-six. There will be a box on the 2015 income tax return regarding whether the person had health insurance for the previous year. Some people filing will need to reconcile the tax credit they received, and those who chose not to obtain coverage and are not eligible for exemption will have to pay a penalty.

The consumer insurance companies are now required to offer and cover preventive services and screening tests like mammograms, cardiac diagnostics, and pregnancy tests. They are banned from placing annual and lifetime limits on benefits, and they are not to allow out-of-pocket payment if expenses exceed the established dollar limits. In addition, insurance companies are now held accountable for an unreasonable rate hike. The elderly on Medicare also can get preventive services paid for and will receive a 50 percent discount on brand-name medications when they reach the "donut hole," or coverage gap. The federal government will subsidize states to add to their Medicaid health program, unless they choose to opt out. There is a marketplace with yearly open enrollment for people to qualify for subsidy or to choose among competing insurance companies. Last but not least, the health-care reform act provides a tax credit for insuring workers at a small business.

One might observe that insurance companies were ahead of

the game. They raised their premiums and dropped several of their insured before Obamacare was implemented. Medicare raised the amount that was deducted from social security beneficiaries.

As our nation embarks on this uncharted path of health care under the Affordable Care Act, there are lots of unanswered questions. How much will Obamacare cost for the insured and the country as a whole? Is preventive care really going to be accessible to everyone? Will new regulations provide care and financial protection to citizens and noncitizens alike? Will medical professionals be able to treat everybody's illnesses, regardless of the patient's income and the treatment's expense? We must also ask whether these provisions and policies are really here to stay, or is the act still in danger of repeal or amendments that change its nature. How long should we prolong life and under what conditions? What benefits will customers be offered and until what age? Related to this, are there going to be any restrictions on any procedures or benefits after a certain age?

The questions continue. Will health insurance companies be exempt from antitrust laws that regulate business corporations, or will there be fair competition for the benefit of consumers? How are administrative costs and claim-processing costs going to be reduced? How is fraud going to be contained? Furthermore, how much waste and abuse will be controlled?

Will Obamacare change over time? If so, how will it be adjusted? Who will be in charge of our health: insurance companies or the government? Will the changes to US health care create a universal health-care system that provides care and financial protection for everybody but that dictates what is covered and for how long? Or will it be a single-payer system, financed and administered by the government? Or it could be a privately delivered health-care system or a combination. Are effective medicines going to be continuously replaced by newer better and more expensive ones? Most importantly, what is our main concern? Are we aiming at health-care finance reform or health-care and wellness reform? In addition, are we pursuing longevity at any cost or promoting wellness and active lifestyles?

Who will decide what preventive and curative benefits are going to be provided? Is the use of expensive technology going to be regulated, and will effective medicines be continuously replaced by newer drugs? How are end-of-life issues going to be handled, particularly considering that the highest cost of health care is incurred during the last few weeks of patient's hospital stay?

Medicine and health care have always been personal topics. During my time as a child, a medical student, and a practicing physician, I have studied medicine; I have also done research and treated patients on three continents. My education and experience gave me a long view on medicine over the centuries. Specialties among the doctors in my family include anesthesiology, cardiology, internal medicine, pathology, pediatrics, surgery (including cancer and vascular surgery), and tropical diseases.

I may not have the answer to all of the aforementioned questions, and I cannot claim that health-care problems are easily solvable. I realize that the big dilemma in health care remains addressing who gets what, why, when, where, how and for how much. However, I can take you through the journey of medicine until the present time and share the external influences on medicine I have seen over the last four decades during practice in the United States and abroad, and I can offer an insider's view of health care. I can reflect on the past; review the changes that have been realized; describe how the art of healing mingled with science; and allude to the effect of automation and information technology on the field of medicine. In addition, I can shed some light on the future of the health-care industry.

I intend to explain the stages medicine went through and

how it changed from the art of observation and interpretation by the doctor—who, in the past, was believed to know best—and became married to science and technology, and then it further transformed into a business wherein the mode of treatment is an informed choice or shared decision between doctor, patient, and insurance company. I may not have answers to all the questions raised, but I might be able to foresee the future of medicine to a degree.

Readers can figure out for themselves what the important factors are in improving the health-care system and decide what changes they would like to be made. They may develop preferences for what is added or deleted from the present version of the Affordable Care Act to lower the cost while improving the care for each individual, emphasizing preventive, diagnostic, and curative measures that need to be implemented.

THOUGHTS FROM THE PAST

All through my life, I have been in close contact with doctors and the medical field. I heard much about medicine; I have studied it, lived it, and practiced it, and I am now reflecting on the past to compare four generations of medical practice. My parents, both physicians, talked a lot about their generation and the previous one, their professors in medical school, with much pride. At that time, Europe—where they studied—and Great Britain were the most advanced countries in medicine as well as many other fields like music art and science.

My mom, the pediatrician, transferred a great deal of knowledge to me during childhood. While tucking me in at bedtime with stories about Little Red Riding Hood, Alice in Wonderland, and Cinderella, she slipped in some of her own life stories. She explained how she rode her bike to the university, the medical school she liked best, and how effectively her professors taught her everything she knew. When I got sick, she treated me with complete bed rest, cold compresses, lots of fluids, lemonade and homemade soup, warm gargles, and aspirin three times a day. She didn't give me antibiotics, for there were none at that time.

My dad, the internist, took over when I was a little older, and he stressed the fun he had studying medicine, how interesting it was to understand the way the human body is built and functions, how rewarding it is to cure a sick person, and how honorable a doctor feels because of his compassion. Their stories were so entertaining and interesting; I was convinced that I should follow in my parents' footsteps and apply to medical school. Only those with the highest grades were accepted, so I worked hard and I was lucky to be one of them. I eventually met my husband there.

When my husband and I went to medical school in Egypt during the late 1940s and early 1950s, most of our professors had been educated in Great Britain. Our medical school followed the British system, and all of our lectures, books, and references were in English even though we lived in an Arabic-speaking country. There was a great emphasis on clinical examination of the patient, and this was a prolonged process. Our instructors taught us to look at the patient's face; you may see pallor, and would therefore need to search for anemia or blood loss. Look into the patient's eyes, and if there's a yellow coloration, test for liver or gallbladder disease, reflected by jaundice; bluish discoloration of the lips can signal hypoxemia (lack of oxygen), a whitish-coated tongue could mean dyspepsia. "Do not hesitate to hold the patients hand," they told us. The person may be cold, or you could feel a rough skin, tremors or discover tender joints or tendons. We followed these observations with examination of the neck, breasts and chest, heart, abdomen, limbs, and so on. Palpation, percussion and auscultation, were our diagnostic means, so touching the patient was important. The first of these methods allowed us to feel enlarged abdominal organs like the spleen, liver, kidney, gallbladder, or any unusual mass; we did not realize that we only would have noticed marked enlargement at a late stage of the disease in question, and there should have been another way for early detection. Percussion was mainly used for chest organs, so an enlarged heart or lung disease could be detected; by tapping the intercostal spaces (between the ribs) all the way from above downward one by one, all over the front and back of the chest, we could differentiate between healthy and diseased lungs. One needed a musical ear. Our teachers explained that this distinction was comparable to testing a watermelon for ripeness: If you tap it and it resonates, it is ripe; if it sounds dull, do not buy it. Similarly, healthy lungs resonate, and dull ones are likely diseased. When performing chest auscultation, it was important to concentrate on hearing a wheeze, indicating bronchial spasm, asthma or partial obstruction, and to listen to a crepitus, meaning the presence of fluid in the lungs. Hearing clear breath sounds at the bases denoted good lung expansion. No medical student or young doctor would go through such a lengthy patient examination at present; it would be a waste of time. At that time, we only ordered x-rays if we felt or heard something unusual, and we only ordered an EKG when heart sounds were abnormal or if we discovered high blood pressure; these procedures were expensive. Routine x-rays and many other advanced diagnostic procedures can now easily show everything we tediously searched for using the senses of vision, hearing, and touch.

Diagnosing an illness was a simple procedure but a tedious, time-consuming one. It relied on the patient's complaint, the medical history and physical exam, a few investigations, the doctor's gut feeling and experience, and maybe one or two laboratory tests or consultations. At the time, the only specialties were general medicine, general surgery (pediatric, cardiac, and vascular surgery were a novelty), OB-GYN (obstetrics and gynecology), ophthalmology, orthopedics, pediatrics, ENT (ear, nose, and throat), dermatology, and cardiopulmonary. Medications and procedures were also limited. Therefore, patient charts consisted of thin, handwritten folders hanging on the person's bed. At the university hospital where we examined patients, they slept side by side in wards of approximately twenty people receiving treatment. There was no privacy at all.

By the time my class graduated, the physician's role was more paternalistic: The doctor said what he or she thought, and the patient listened and acquiesced totally to the doctor, whom the whole family knew, trusted, and never questioned. This physician would have been the family doctor for decades. They visited a doctor in the office, or he or she made house calls, depending on the severity of the patient's sickness. The family paid the physician in cash on the spot, and the doctor decided the fee for the service he provided, no questions asked. Bargaining would have happened rarely, because the doctor was the life saver, not to be argued with. Health care was affordable and easy to maintain during that time period.

Although medical school required several years of hard work, we experienced funny things that gave our lives levity. For example, patients scheduled for surgery and on NPO, or nothing by mouth, instructions hid food in their nightstands, believing that eating the evening before surgery would give them more strength to get over the anesthesia. When they did this, the surgery had to be rescheduled, and nurses had to thoroughly search for hidden food. There was a particular patient in the dermatology department whom we all talked about for many years. Psoriasis was a common skin disease, and its treatment was limited to white ointment (zinc oxide) or black ointment (tar). This patient got bored indoors and walked all over the hospital yard half naked, painted white or black; we called him Frankenstein, and because his disease was chronic, he was continually in and out of the hospital. He was there when we were students, interns, and residents, with no improvement in his condition or innovation regarding his treatment. Although we made fun of him his condition was pitiful but we could do nothing about it.

Other chronic patients we saw during our rounds included young adults with rheumatic fever and those with complicated heart disease, with or without heart failure. These same patients were the subjects of our clinical exams at the end of the year. They were aware of their own symptoms, and they gave us hints like telling us to listen to a "diastolic murmur on the second intercostal space," or they said, "There is a systolic murmur at the apex," "I have fibrillation," or "My blood pressure is so-and-so," or "Feel my pulse it is irregular,"or "Examine my abdomen I have an enlarged liver and spleen."They gave us their diagnosis in English, even though they did not speak the language. In other words, they were poor and ignorant yet smart enough to memorize what their doctors discussed among themselves. Of course, we still examined each patient thoroughly and made sure that what they recited was correct; sure enough, many times it was. Every once in a while, one of the more able chronic patients took the liberty of joining the intern or resident making his or her rounds as an aid—for example, handing the doctor the sphygmomanometer (to measure blood pressure), thermometer, or patient's chart if the nurse was busy.

Sometimes discharged patients came back to visit their friends and smuggled things to those still in treatment that they were not medically allowed to have in the hospital. There were also illiterate patients who came from neighboring villages to be treated for free at the university hospital, desperate after not improving under the care of their local physician. They were the most difficult to examine, as it was impossible to get any meaningful disease history or an accurate description of their complaint. Frequently, they misled us by telling us symptoms they heard from a neighbor or a friend who felt better taking a certain medication and requesting the same, not their own symptoms, thinking the same treatment would help them. I remember how surprised I was when I asked a lady what her complaint was before I started to examine her, and she said that her children were her biggest problem; they just don't listen. I asked another patient when the pain started, and she answered that it was when she moved out. I inquired further about when she moved out. She told me that it was when her youngest quit school. "Okay, and when was that?" I prompted.

"Sometime last year," she finally said.

There was no way to get a definite answer.

Patients also exaggerated pain to get more sympathy and attention. They commonly said, "It is all over my body and hurts severely; I cannot pinpoint a single area." No matter how frustrating that was, we made fun of such incidents, and we still remember them and laugh. However, it saddened us to realize how poverty and lack of education can negatively affect people's health.

Another unforgettable funny incident involved a well-trained doctor. As students, we were required to watch some surgeries while they were performed. The anesthesiologist prepared the patient while the surgeon scrubbed and got gowned. At the time, patients inhaled gases like ether to reach anesthesia, while counting till falling asleep; it usually only took a count to ten. In this instance, when the surgeon was ready to start, he heard the patient still counting: "Two hundred, two hundred one, two hundred two ..." He awoke the poor anesthesiologist who had been on call the night before and make him aware that his patient was not under yet and remind him to watch the dosage. Instead of surgical methods, we learned from this incident that a health-care professional must be healthy and alert.

When my peers and I started to work, the major difference between the way our generation practiced medicine and my parents' generation practiced it involved using newer medications few innovations in techniques and procedures as well as some more specializations. These minor changes prompted many competitive discussions between us, a situation that brought back memories of my parents' schooling. We talked about our progress and innovations, they told many stories about the medical schools they attended and the extraordinary teachers who taught them, who were researchers, discoverers, and scientists, and stressed that many among them were pioneers in their fields. My parents explained that during those days in Germany, students moved from one university to another to study under the best professor in a particular subject. For example, some specialties were better taught in Hamburg; other professors were considered more advanced in their subjects in Leipzig; basic sciences were strongest in Heidelberg; and other fields were best in Munich or Berlin. My parents' certification of graduation included all of these universities.

They talked about Heidelberg University (figure 1) and the students there; some of them proudly showed off the scars they had obtained from the sport of fencing. The university was founded in 1386, and it was the hub for independent thinkers. It served as a role model to other schools, and it still attracts many foreign students for postgraduate studies, with approximately one thousand doctoral degrees given every year. Twenty percent of its student body is made up of international students from one hundred thirty countries. In 2008, Heidelberg University was ranked first in Germany, fourth in Europe, and thirteenth in the world

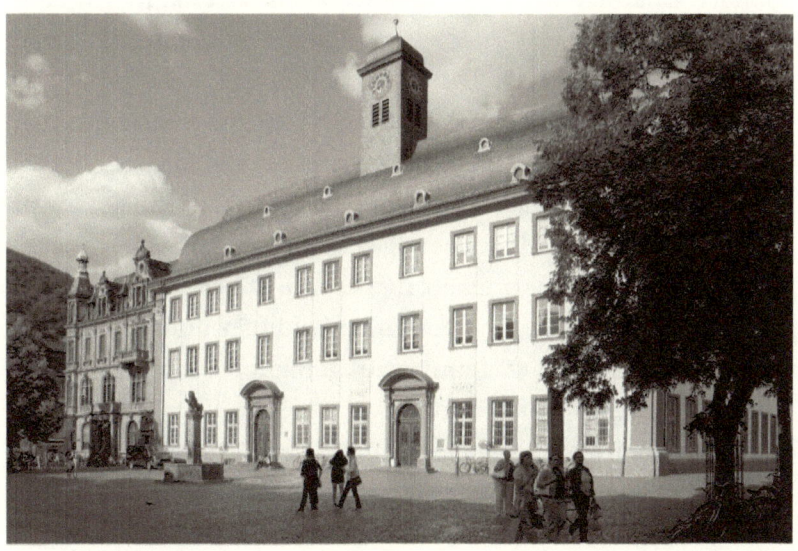

FIGURE 1

by the number of its Nobel Laureates. Fifty-five Nobel Prizes have been granted to researchers connected with the university. Today, it consists of twelve faculties and offers undergraduate, graduate, and postdoctoral programs. It is well known for its botanical garden, for being one of the oldest places of study in the world for pharmaceutics, and for its chemical laboratory. When I visited Heidelberg University in 1964, I found it located in a charming and beautiful old town. In fact, the Old Town campus is situated in the pedestrian zone of the University Square, and every visitor walking through the downtown area can enjoy its views while listening to the church bells ringing on every hour.

The new university, which officially opened its doors in 1931, was largely financed by wealthy American families such as Goldman, Sachs, Morgan, Chrysler, and Ford. Marcus Goldman was born in Germany and started his business in New York, in the United States, in 1869. His son-in-law, Samuel Sacks, joined him in 1882, and Goldman's son joined in 1885. Together, they founded Goldman Sachs and adopted its present name. The company became famous for pioneering the use of commercial paper for entrepreneurs and was invited to join the New York Stock Exchange (NYSE). Henry Morgan and Harold Stanley started their business with J. P. Morgan and then split off and formed Morgan Stanley. Walter Chrysler and Henry Ford are well known for pioneering their automobile manufacturing companies in the early 1900s. Those generous philanthropists recognized the significance of health care, science, and education, and they donated much of their money to keep this university going for a long time as an important scientific institution.

When we lived in Heidelberg in 1963 and 1964 and revisited it in 1968, it was a small old city compared to other cities we visited in Germany, which were more modern and much more developed. A story goes that during the Second World War, the American pilot who was sent to bombard the region intentionally missed Heidelberg because he had visited it before, in the early 1930s; he was fascinated with its architecture and fell in love with it. The city, therefore, was not destroyed during the war like most other German cities; they needed to be rebuilt and thus modernized after the war, but Heidelberg retained its beautiful old architecture thanks to an American pilot.

My dad frequently mentioned the University of Munich. It is considered one of the most prestigious universities in Europe. He never failed to say that when he studied there, he and his colleagues enjoyed going for a big mug of beer and attended the Oktoberfest the city is famous for. The university was founded in 1472 but moved twice till it settled in its present location in 1826 with the help of prince Maximillian IV and King Ludwig I of Bavaria. The institution is well known for Professor Wilhelm Rontgen and his invention of x-rays as well as for Ferdinand Sauerbruch, professor of surgery. My parents talked about him with pride; they went to Munich especially to attend his lectures. My parents told me that this professor was born in the city of Barmen in 1875. His grandfather raised him because of his dad's early death, and then he studied medicine in Gottingen and started practicing in 1901. In 1904 he established the ground rules for thoracic surgery, including how to prevent the collapse of the lungs during the procedure, by developing the pressure chamber for operating on the chest, thus counteracting negative pressure in the chest cavity. In 1907, Sauerbruch worked on the possibilities and boundaries of organ transplant. During the period from 1910 to 1918, he put together steps for surgical interference for pulmonary tuberculosis, and in 1915, he developed the Sauerbruch Hand, a device to facilitate the musculoskeletal (muscle-and-bone) system in improving hand movement. In 1928, when he became professor of surgery in Berlin, his colleagues dubbed him "Der Chirurg," or "the surgeon." It is no secret that he lived and suffered much through the Nazi era, and he protested against euthanasia. Professor Sauerbruch passed away in 1951, yet in my parent's thoughts, he lived forever. His family produced leaders and pioneers in different fields; his son was a well-known painter, and his grandson was a leader in architecture. This talented family also included innovators, artists, and scientists.

Another school my parents talked about a lot was the University of Hamburg, established in 1919. Because of the city's location close to the harbor on the river Elbe, close to its mouth at the North Sea, and because it had the third busiest port in the world at that time, the Bernard Nocht Institute for Tropical Medicine was established there. The doctors there examined and treated sailors and other travelers near Hamburg's port, coming from countries where tropical diseases were known to be endemic. My father got his doctoral degree from this institution in the late 1920s, and I visited it on a fellowship in 1963. To reach the institute, one went down Reeperbahn Street, meaning "rope walk," in St. Paulo: one of two big centers for night life, where sailors spent their evenings. I was shocked by the number of nightclubs, restaurants, discos, and strip clubs on this street and surprised by the way they used their windows for advertisement. For many years, this school was considered the leading institute for researchers to learn about tropical diseases in a non- tropical country, and I learned several new ways of testing for tropical diseases during my work in their labs, I was able to apply when I returned to treat patients in my country.

The second-oldest university in Germany, which was in Leipzig, Saxon, had one of the best medical schools. It was better known for producing philosophers like Nietzsche and Goethe, who was also a writer; artists; and musicians like Wagner. Unfortunately, it deteriorated after World War II, for it became part of East Germany. It was revived later, when East and West Germany reunited. This university has one of the most important pharmacology institutions.

Although I never visited it, I can relate to it, because my mother was born there and lived there.

It is quite interesting to think of the big differences in practice between these past two generations, my parents and their professors; my own generation (the third); and now our children's generation (the fourth). It is truly amazing to see how much progress was made in the medical field during the twentieth century, but I can also attest to some disadvantages as patterns for practicing medicine have changed over the years. I have witnessed the practice of medicine in three different continents: Africa, Europe, and North America, during different decades; this made it an even more interesting subject to write about.

When I graduated in the mid-1950s, my interest was to specialize in tropical medicine and start my career on the medical staff of the university hospital. According to the British system, I needed a diploma in internal medicine, followed by a diploma in tropical medicine and a doctoral degree. I was interested in the diseases affecting that part of the world, particularly the endemic ones that were seldom seen in colder weather and in countries with better hygiene standards. Some diseases caused by worms and parasites include ascariasis, ameabiasis, ankylostomiasis, filariasis, trichinosis, and malaria. In addition to other problems they all cause nutritional deficiency and anemia; the primary one was schistosomiasis, also known as bilharzia. Some believe that this disease was the main reason Ancient Egyptians did not live longer than thirty-five years. The Ebers Papyrus, an old Egyptian document, addressed symptoms of this disease as well as its treatment and how to prevent the bleeding it caused. It has always been mentioned that it was difficult to believe that one could contract such a deadly disease from the water in a country considered to be the gift of the Nile River. The cause of death was bleeding or kidney disease and bladder cancer. Another old Egyptian document, the Hearst Papyrus, mentions using the chemical compound antimony disulfide as a remedy; amazingly enough, we used injections of this same compound centuries later in spite of its severe toxic side effects. Only during my residency, other medications that were more effective and less hazardous were being researched and implemented.

Bilharzia was the topic of my doctoral degree, and I researched it thoroughly. It was of utmost interest to me when I found out that Theodor Maximillian Bilharz (March 23, 1825–May 9, 1862), after whom the disease was named, was a German physician who graduated from Tubingen University in 1848 and was chief of pathology at the University of Freiburg. He went to Egypt in 1850 at the time of the ruler Abbas the First to study insects and parasites, and he occupied three positions there: chief of surgery, medical consultant, and served in the military as a kaimakam lieutenant colonel. Unfortunately, his passion killed him. He died in the Red Sea region in 1862 of typhus, an insect-born disease, at the age of thirty-seven and was buried in Cairo. During his short stay in Egypt working at Kasr El Eini hospital, he discovered a worm he called schistosoma, for it had a split body; the worm name was later changed to Bilharzia in his honor. During the early 1900s, other researchers discovered the very interesting worm's life cycle and that the worm's larvae caused the disease, by piercing the patient's skin and they were transmitted by snails living along the banks of the Nile (figure 2.)

In the early 1960s, The Theodor Bilharz Research Institute in Giza was named after him, for the great discovery he made.

We completely devoted six and a half years of our lives to medical school. During the first three, we were mainly consumed with basic science, chemistry, histology, anatomy, pharmacology, reading books, and researching references as well as running many experiments in the labs; the last three and a half years, we were absorbed in clinical departments, lectures and patient examination.

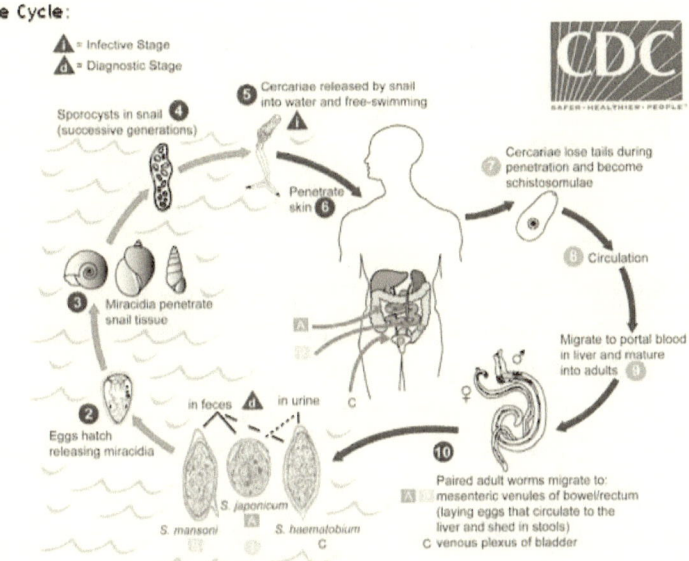

FIGURE 2

After graduation from medical school but before starting to practice, we were required to familiarize ourselves with the Hippocratic oath (figure 3), the rule of ethics in medicine. The oath originated in Greece and has been translated to many languages. Each newly graduated physician at that time had to swear upon a number of gods that he or she would uphold a number of professional ethical standards that bound student to teacher, community, and peers with responsibilities similar to that of a family member. There are several versions of the translations, but the most prominent is as follows:

> *I swear by Apollo the physician, and Hygeia and panacea and all the gods and goddesses as my witnesses, that, according to my ability and judgment, I will keep this Oath and this contract:*
> *To hold him who taught me this art equally dear to me as my parents, to be partner in life with him, and*

to fulfill his needs when required; to look upon his off-spring as equals to my own siblings, and to teach
them this art, if they shall wish to learn it, without fee or contract; and that by the set rules, lectures, and every other mode of instruction, I will impart a knowledge of the art to my own sons, and those of my teachers, and to students bound by this contract and having sworn this Oath to the law of medicine, but to no others.
I will use those dietary regimens which will benefit my patients according to my greatest ability and judgment, and will do no harm or injustice to them
I will not give a lethal drug to anyone if I am asked, nor will I advise such a plan; and similarly I will not give a woman a pessary to cause abortion.
In purity and according to divine law will I carry out my life and my art.
I will not use the knife, even upon those suffering from stones, but I will leave this to those who are trained in this craft
Into whatever homes I go, I will enter them for the benefit of the sick, avoiding any voluntary act of impropriety or corruption, including the seduction of women or men, whether they are free men or slaves. Whatever I see or hear in the lives of my patients, whether in connection with my professional practice or not, which ought not to be spoken of outside, I will keep secret, as considering all such things to be private. So long as I maintain this Oath faithfully and without corruption, may it be granted to me to partake of life fully and the practice of my art, gaining the respect of all men for all time. However should I transgress this Oath and violate it, may the opposite be my fate.

"Twelfth-century Byzantine manuscript the oath was written out in the form of a cross, relating it visually to Christian ideas".

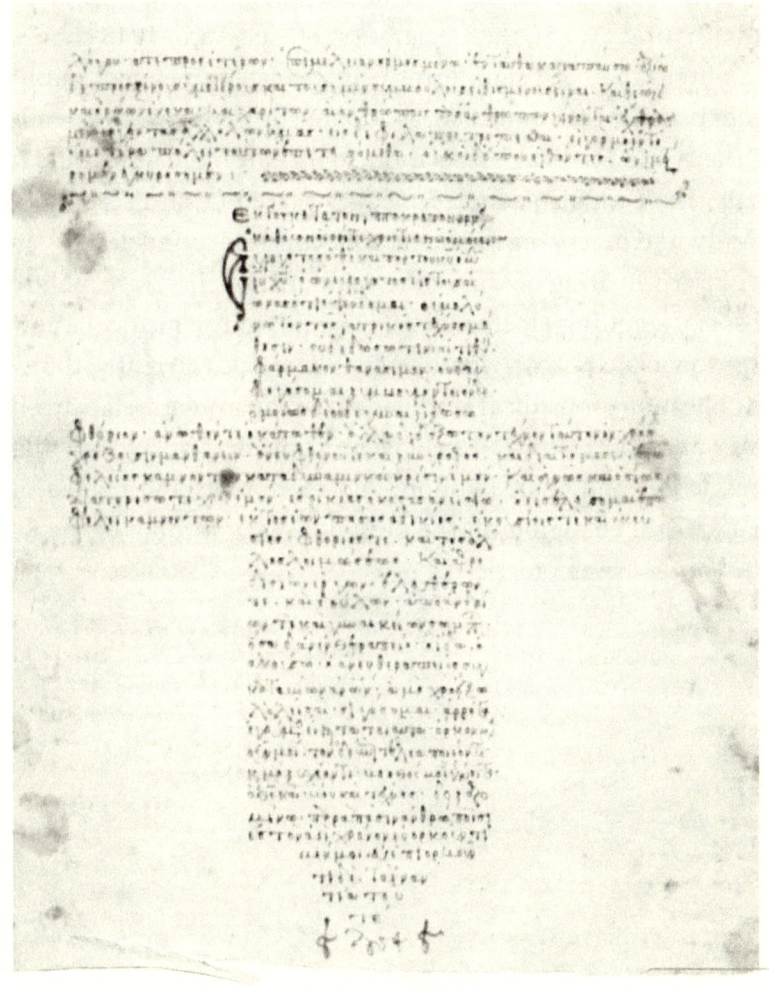

FIGURE 3

The oath demonstrates that physicians cherished their job and how seriously they felt about the art of healing and the craft of surgery in ancient times. Needless to say, doctors on later centuries swore to the one Christian, Jewish and Moslem God rather than Apollo. The oath has been modified several times and in many different countries throughout its existence, and after the atrocities of World War II, the Declaration of Geneva in 1948 changed the physician's oath significantly. It was later amended multiple times between1968 and 2006, as adopted by the General Assembly of The World Medical Association, to include more humanitarian goals. The oath also adopted pledges geared toward serving humanity, and practicing medicine with conscience and dignity, and not discriminating because of religion, nationality, race, politics, or social standing; doctors also swore not to use medical knowledge to violate human rights or civil liberties. Currently, there is no obligation for medical graduates to swear any oath; statistically, fewer and fewer do, yet I believe most of them still follow their consciences and abide by more and more rules and regulations that are still changing till the present time according to the way medicine is being practiced.

ANCIENT HISTORY

I was born in Egypt and lived there for about one third of my life; I am proud to be an Egyptian American, and I am proud of my ancestors who were well-known pioneers in [AlGabr] algebra, [AlChemia] chemistry, architecture, astronomy, and medicine. I went to elementary school, high school, and medical school there; I studied and read books by respected authors that familiarized me with the country's ancient history, and I visited its archeological wonders and cultural museums while I was growing up. My husband and I went back to visit in 1997 with our son and his wife, both physicians; they were interested to see firsthand the art of healing, how it started in ancient civilization and how medicine developed into what they had recently studied and are now practicing. We had a few good days visiting with family and old friends and a relaxing time along the beautiful Mediterranean beaches neighboring Alexandria as well as those in Sharm and Hurghada at the Red Sea. Most importantly, we took a long tour, starting in Cairo. We visited the archeological sites at the tombs of Giza and the pyramids of Saqqara, and we took the Nile cruise to Upper Egypt, disembarking on the way in several cities passing through all the temples there, most notably the one in Luxor. The information we obtained from the displays in museums and the writing on the walls of temples was extremely educational.

It is said that if one had to be ill in ancient times, Egypt would probably have been the best place to be. Ancient Egyptians believed that sickness was a mystery and the work

of an evil-spirited god, and that prayers to Sekhmet the goddess of healing was the cure. The priest-physician used magic
to treat patients but also advised them about a healthy diet and
prescribed herbal medicines; surprisingly, they were the same
herbs that have been rediscovered recently and are presently
in vogue. Ancient Egyptians used garlic, which is said to lower
cholesterol and blood pressure; they peeled, mashed, and
mixed cloves with vinegar and water, and used this concoction
as mouthwash. Coriander was indicated to cure indigestion
and to prevent excessive gas and bloating. Cumin, an herb
indigenous to Egypt, was mixed with coriander, and this combination seemed to be effective in preventing flatulence.
Drinking a pomegranate infusion was prescribed to get rid of
some intestinal parasites; castor oil, figs, and dates relieved
constipation; tannic acid derived from acacia nuts was used to
relieve burns, and henna was grown and used to prevent hair
loss by men and women. We also discovered that hashish and
opium were used for relaxation and to alleviate pain. Looking
at illustrations of ancient Egyptians, we noticed that the pre-
dominant type of makeup was eyeliner. This is because they
used malachite as a therapeutic and preventive measure for eye
infections such as trachoma, which was endemic even in ancient times. In addition to herbal medicines, they treated ach-
ing limbs by massaging them with mud. Because healers were
priests and doctors, temples were equipped with examination
areas and laboratories (pharmacies) where they prepared and
stored medicines. Papyrus documents were the main source of
this information and much more about medicine in Egypt
from 1900 to 1500 BC.

An American archeologist purchased the Ebers Papyrus 1550,
(figure 4), approximately twenty meters long and third of a me-
ter wide, from an Egyptian in 1862. It contains about 110 pages,

and it is the most recent known papyrus, written in the hieratic Egyptian language; translations from this language were possible after the discovery of the Rosetta Stone. The papyrus references the reign of Amhotep, known to be the oldest physician (1725 BC). He was influential enough to commission a pyramid to be built for himself, and he was also an astrologer. He was said to be

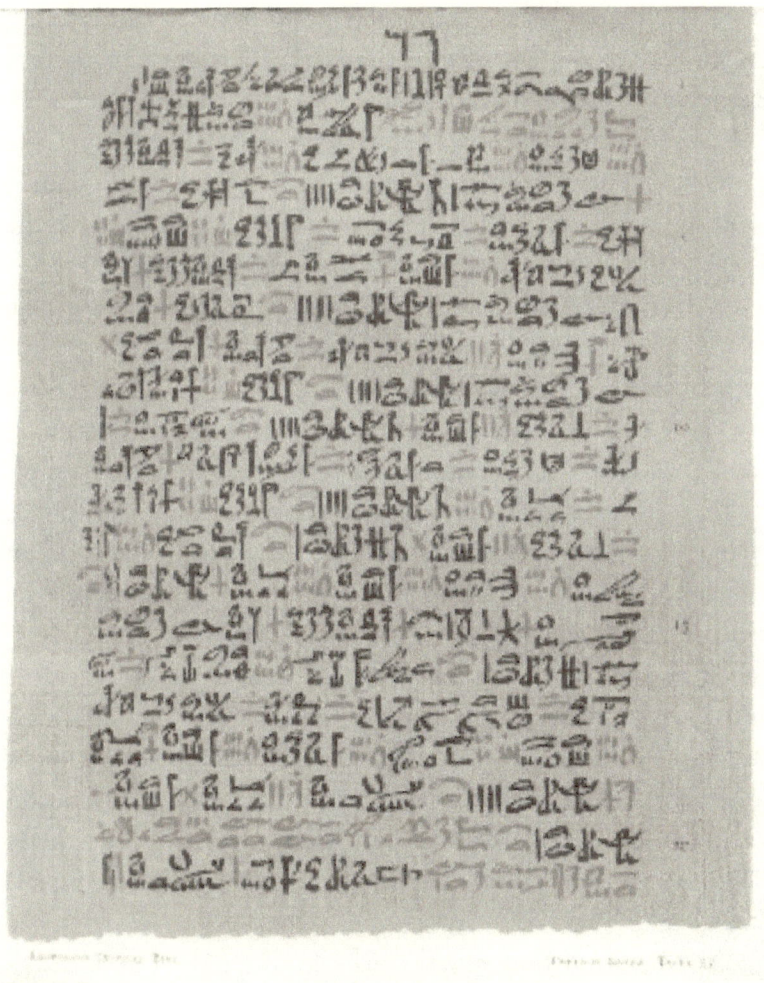

FIGURE 4

the physician of the King Zoser; after his death, people worshiped him as a god because of their faith in his power to cure sickness. The Ebers Papyrus also contained references to the heart, blood vessels, stomach and intestinal ailments, skin conditions, and ear and nose infections; there was also some mention of organs like the spleen and lungs and mental conditions. Surprisingly, the document even describes eight cases of tumors of the breast to which there was no cure, probably referring to cancer, and it recommended cauterization of the mass. There are actually seven Egyptian papyri, written between 3000 and 1500 BC, describing diseases that could be nowadays diagnosed as cancer.

Egyptologist Edwin Smith brought the Edwin Smith papyrus 1600, named after him (figure 5) from Luxor, Egypt, to the United States before Ebers arrived with his. An Egyptian vendor sold it to Smith in 1822, and it was only translated from hieroglyphics in 1930. Dr. Robert Wilkins of Duke University referred to it and considered it a neurosurgical classic. It is now in the Cyber Museum of Neurosurgery, and it is part of the collections of the New York Academy of Science. This papyrus is one of the oldest-known medical documents revealing surgical cases that are systematically organized, starting with injuries to the head and proceeding downward anatomically through the body. They were organized into the categories treatable, uncertain, and unfavorable, the latter meaning "untreatable." It is remarkably detailed, describing the cranial structures of the bony skull and brain surface, the covering, and the fluid within as well as the relation between brain injuries and other functions of the body. It is second in length to the Ebers Papyrus and consists of seventeen pages, 377 lines, on the right side and five pages and ninety-two lines on the left side.

It is believed that much of the knowledge of anatomy by Ancient Egyptians arose from the process of mummification, which was performed in a scientific and sophisticated manner. First, those performing mummification removed the brain by suction through the nose, and other internal organs, and then they dehydrated the body for forty days using natron, a mixture of salts, they knew that humidity would make the corpse more liable to rot. Next, they stuffed the body cavity with linen and sawdust and painted the skin with herbal preparations, coated it with resin, and wrapped it in linen. This procedure taught them the exact positions of every organ in the body cavity.

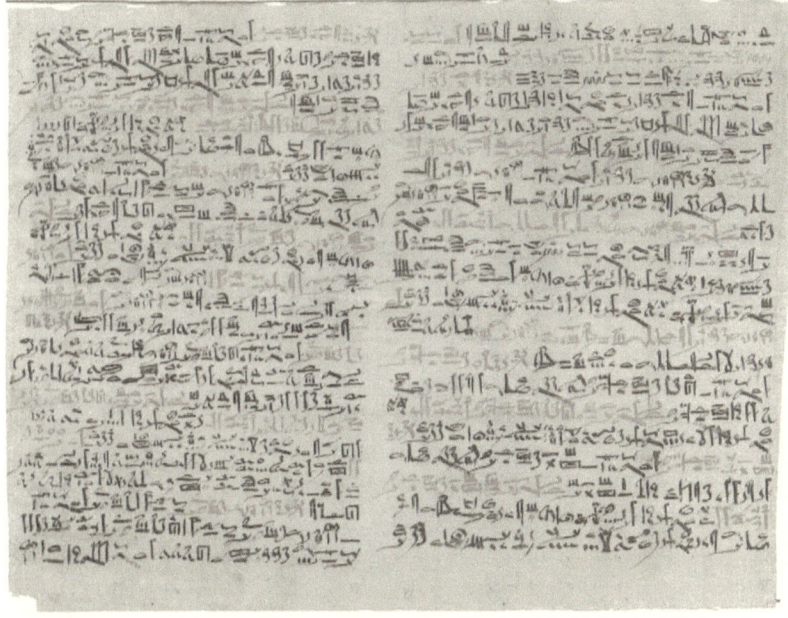

FIGURE 5

There are smaller and less significant documents of papyrus, such as the Hearst Papyrus, dated to the Eighteenth Dynasty, around the time of Pharaoh Tuhotmus; it contains remedial methods and medications for different ailments. The Kahun Papyrus, discovered by Flinders Patria in 1889 in the city of Fayum, is dated to the reign of Amenemhat II and translated into English by Griffin in 1898. It resides at the London University College and is mainly gynecological in subject matter. The Berlin Papyrus 6619 is another document from the Middle Kingdom, found in the ancient burial ground of Saqqara in the early nineteenth century CE, it contains obstetric and gynecological information and it documents the use of pregnancy testing. The publication by Hans Schackenburg in 1900 indicates that it was also the primary source of Ancient Egyptian Mathematics. Also at Saqqara is the tomb of Ankh-Mahor, or the tomb of the physician; the images on its walls depict different minor surgeries (Figure 6).

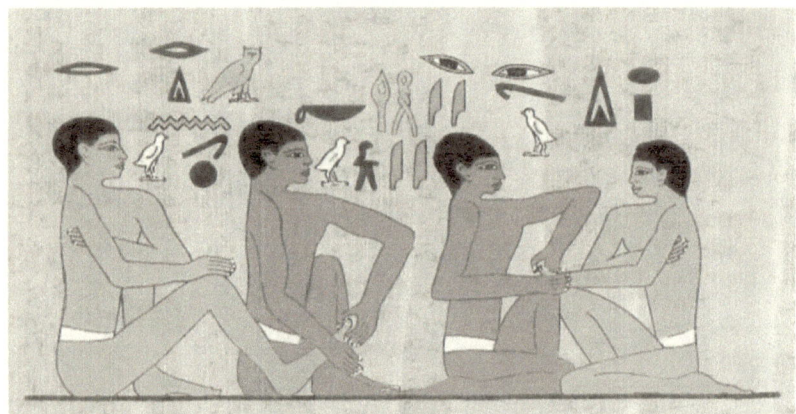

FIGURE 6

During our tours, the guide explained that some of the archeological findings represented pictures of medical practices and names of doctors and their various specialties. On a wall of the Temple of Kom Ombo, there is a carved relief of a box of surgical instruments; it contains shears, surgical knives, saws, probes, spatula, hooks, and forceps; thirty-seven types of tools are engraved on one wall. Similar illustrations are also present in the museum of Cairo. Egyptian instruments were mostly made of copper—an improvement from earlier ones that had stone blades—flint, surgical steel, and bronze or iron. Reliefs of medical instruments like dental tools, bone saws, scales, lances, suction cups, and retractors also appear in the temple of Sobek.

A display of surgical instruments from Ancient Rome, originally excavated from a Pompeii surgeon's house and exhibited at the health science library at the University of Virginia, represents a collection of the tools at the disposal of surgeons in the first century BCE. It demonstrates that there was very little innovation since the time of Hippocrates (fifth century BCE) and Galen (second century CE. Therefore, it represents the instruments used in surgery for nearly a millennium with no improvements or additions, and it includes similar specula, levers, forceps, cupping vessels (for bloodletting), cautery, probes, catheters, osteotomes (for bone cutting), scalpels, scissors, and curettes to those seen in the Egyptian tombs.

The earliest report of surgical suture material was in ancient Egypt, circa 3000 BC, and it was made from flax, hemp, or cotton, animal tendon strips and muscle strips, or silk. Galen described gut suture from sheep intestine as "catgut." I remember using this material during training. We used to joke about introducing it into the human body; we assumed it was obtained from cats. He also discussed straight and curved needles used to suture, some with an eye and the suture material threaded through it, and eyeless ones with suture material preattached; each had a specific indication. Unfortunately, they all frequently produced wound infections and delayed recovery till the early 1930s, with the introduction of absorbable suture material based on polyvinyl alcohol and nonabsorbable chemically produced polyester suture material, customized for different layers of skin and internal organs. Our tour of Egypt lasted eighteen days, during which time we gained much knowledge about the history of medicine and its practice considered to be an art of healing there over the centuries.

By the year 1200 BC, when Greece became more advanced in farming, warfare, sailing, and craftsmanship, there was also a big turn in medicine. Its famous doctor, Hippocrates, became extremely famous in medicine as he tried to find a natural explanation for why people got sick and died. Ailed individuals used to go to temples to seek the help of the god Apollo. Hippocrates, credited as the father of western medicine, thought of medicine as a discipline distinct from fields it was associated with before like magic and philosophy; his idea was that it should be a separate profession and therefore established his own medical school and the corpus was attributed to him and his medical students. The first known Greek medical school, however, was established in 700 BC, during the archaic period. The Greeks imported a lot of medical knowledge from Egypt during the period when Ptolemy made advances in biology; he located intelligence in the brain and showed the connection of the nervous system to motion and sensation. The imported knowledge from Egypt also included additions to their pharmacopoeia; this influence became more pronounced after the establishment of a school of medicine in Alexandria, Egypt, after Alexander the Great invaded it around 300 BC. The famous library at Alexandria housed the collection of writings attributed to Hippocrates, known as the Hippocratic corpus (Figure 7), where he categorized illnesses into acute; chronic long-standing; endemic, deeply rooted in the country; and epidemic, widespread. He explained exacerbations and relapses of the same disease. Claudius Galen also studied in Alexandria; he was born in Turkey, of Greek parents, and then he moved to Rome in the early 160s CE, lived there and became the physician to the Emperor. He was the most famous doctor in the Roman Empire and he originated experimental medical investigation. He was

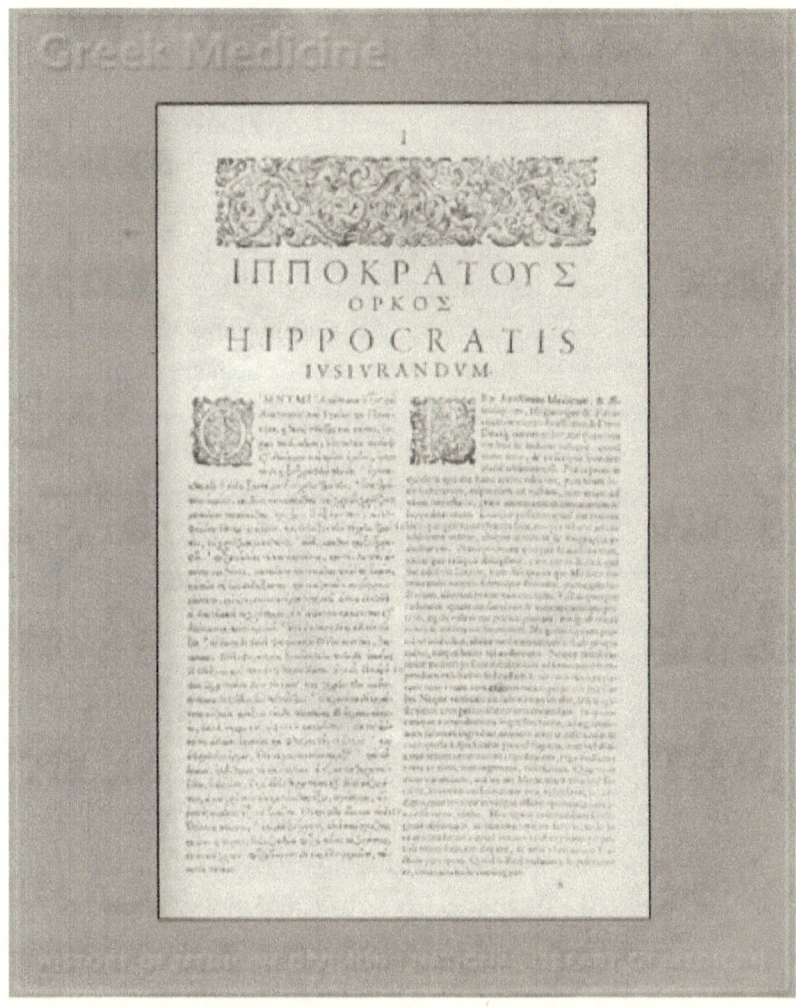

FIGURE 7

interested in studying the body's anatomy and functions and is said to have performed many animal dissections to find out what occurs inside the body. He could prove that urine was formed in the kidneys and that blood ran in arteries.

Later, during the Middle Ages in Europe, the Roman Catholic Church proclaimed that sickness was punishment from God to sinners; to argue against this concept was considered heresy, so Greek-based medicine stagnated till about the fourteenth century CE. Even so, there was a turning point during the period from 500 BC to 146 CE, when the Roman Empire grew and took over part of Greece. They learned a lot and applied the knowledge, and they concentrated more on improving the quality of life for the entire population rather than only curing the sick. They were under the impression that poor hygiene, unclean water, and sewage caused illness. Therefore, they dealt with the public health system, public water supply, and drainage systems, and they built toilets not only for the rich but also for the poor. Wherever they built new settlements, they constructed public baths. They also believed that to stay healthy, one needed to stay fit, so they encouraged athletics.

The Islamic Golden Age (661–750 CE) flourished during the reign of the Abbasid Caliphate. Islamic medicine had a Greco-Roman background, yet when Islam spread from the Arabian Peninsula (from the mid seventh to the 13th century), its civilization extended from India in the east to the Atlantic Ocean in the west. It spread easily because of the unified Arabic language at the time to simplify reading the Koran and the fairness of the rulers. Its effect was most obvious in Spain (Andalusia), throughout many cities like Granada, Cordoba, and Seville, sometime between 800 and 1450 CE. Persia, which became part of the Islamic world in 636, also became a hub. In the capital, Gundeshapur, a big medical school opened and became the greatest center for medical teaching for the following two hundred years.

There are many writings that refer to the Arab roots of European medicine and the contributions of physicians of Arab origin to the art of healing. Even the *Canterbury Tales*, written in Middle English by Geoffrey Chaucer (1342–1400) about pilgrims telling stories while travelling together during the hundred year war, refers to the most popular doctors of Islam as great authorities in medicine. The verses were later translated into modern English by "Ronald L Ecker and Eugene J Crook". The verses go as follows:

> *Well Knew he the olde Esculapius*
> *And Deyscadides and eek Rufus*
> *Olde Ypocras, Haly and Galeyn*
> *Sevapion, Razi and Avycen*
> *Averrois, Damascien and Constantyn*
> *Bernard, and Gatesden and Gilbertyn.*

The Abbasid Caliphate realized the importance of the Greek medical works and established a translation bureau in Baghdad. Hunayn ibn Ishaq al Ibadi carried out translation into Arabic; he was reportedly paid for his work on manuscripts by their weight in gold. The bureau translated the entire body of Greek medical texts by Galen, Oribasins, and Hippocrates as well as *De materia medica* (figure 8), the collective knowledge at the time about the therapeutic properties of any substance used for healing medicines, put together by Pedanius Dioscorides. It mainly contained plants and their extracts, (figure 9).

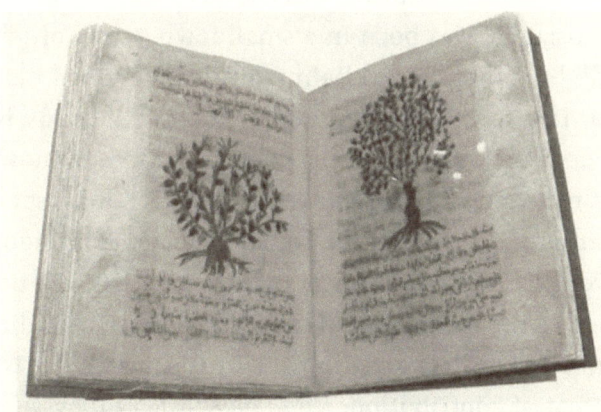

FIGURE 8

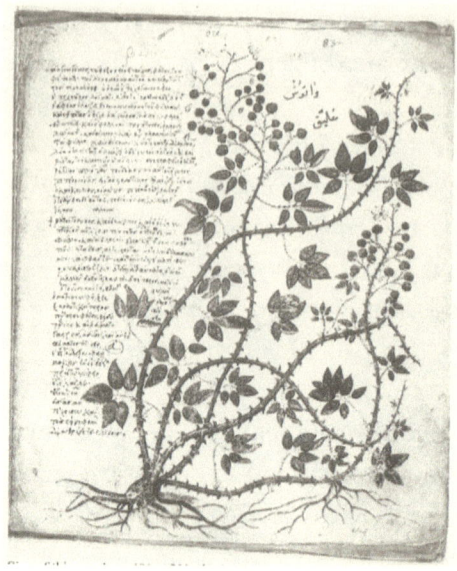

FIGURE 9

This branch of science is now referred to as pharmacology; Jabir ibn Hayyan was considered the father of Arab chemistry because he composed the first pharmacological treatises in the world.

Abu al-Qasim al-Zahrawi was another Arab scholar who lived in Andalusia. He was born in a small town near Cordoba, built in 936 CE by Caliph Abdul Rahman III, who named Zahra after Zahrawi. This scholar, known in the West as Albucasis, is said to have made spectacular advances in surgery and was known as the father of modern surgery; he invented the anesthetic sponge that contained a mixture of opium, Indian hemp, and belladonna. He also developed modern surgical instrumentation. His books are still found in the International Institute of Islamic Medicine and the Islamic Medical Association of North America. He is famous for his greatest contribution, *Kitab al-Tasrif*, a thirty-volume encyclopedia of medical practice, distributed all over the world, containing methods for treating all diseases and a pharmacopeia. Abu al-Qasim al-Zahrawi is also known for documenting the first reliable description of a successful thyroidectomy, dating back to the tenth century CE. Under opium sedation, he removed a large goiter—that is, an enlarged thyroid gland, from a man who was seated with a large bag around his neck to catch the blood flowing from the neck incision. During the 1700s and early 1800s, thyroid surgery was banned; it was thought to be barbaric and horrid butchery because it caused severe hemorrhaging and infection with a mortality rate up to 40 percent. Between 1877 and 1880, Theodore Billroth and Theodore Kocher revived the surgery by popularizing the Kocher incision of the neck, which reduced bleeding and brought the mortality rate down to 1 percent.

Albucasis was also the first surgeon to describe ectopic, or extra-uterine, pregnancy as well as identifying the hereditary nature of hemophilia, a blood disease causing extensive bleeding only in male offspring from mothers carrying the gene. In his books, he described the instruments and techniques that he invented for surgery. The Abbasids were influenced by the Koranic injunction that stressed the value of knowledge; because they believed that Allah has a cure for every sickness, it was their duty to keep researching till they found the answer to every problem. Therefore, Islamic medicine flourished from the eighth century to the fifteenth century while Europe was still in the Dark Ages, "A period of intellectual darkness, barbarity, and economic regression that occurred after the collapse of the Western Roman Empire." Charitable donations were paid for new hospitals across the Islamic world, and there was a stress on educating physicians by the tutorial system. Medical literature was integrated with natural science, astrology, chemistry, philosophy, and religion.

Mohamed Ibn Zakariya al-Razi (865–925 CE) was another well-known Persian physician during the Islamic Golden Age. He was multitalented, interested in science, music, chemistry, mathematics, metaphysics, and philosophy, but he went to Baghdad at the age of forty to study medicine for his career. He was known as the father of pediatrics. Among the more than hundred books he wrote, the most important was his treatise on children's diseases. He made many contributions to medical research, clinical care, and use of chemicals. His prominence was based on his honesty, a belief in ethics, and a stress on morality; he tried to differentiate between curable and incurable diseases. Al-Razi was a proponent of experimental medicine and a leader in fighting witchcraft. He trained in Greek philosophy and studied medicine under Ali El Tabari, the Muslim hakim (physician and psychologist) who was known to help the poor and combined philosophy and medicine in his writings. He (al-Razi) issued the great medical compendium and was also the first to differentiate between smallpox and measles.

The prominent philosopher of the Islamic era, Ibn-Sina—known in the West as Avicenna—compiled the *Quanun fi al Tib*, the law of medicine, as an encyclopedia of five books, completing it in 1025 CE. It presented an organized summary of all medical knowledge of the time, and it stressed the importance of diet and the influence of the environment on people's health; the work was originally written in Arabic and translated into numerous languages. Its principles were treated as the bible of medicine for a long time, and although that was centuries ago, it is still taught at UCLA and Yale University as part of medical history. Since I went to medical school in Egypt and then trained at UCLA when I moved to the United States, I am well aware of Ibn-Sina's contributions to medicine. I was also lucky enough to be able to read this treasure in its original language.

Ibn-Sina was a legend. At the age of ten, he completely memorized the Koran; he then studied law, physics, mathematics, and philosophy. At the age of sixteen, he started to study medicine, and by twenty, he was appointed as a court physician and later became vizier, or minister; later in his life, he was dedicated to writing. *The Book of Healing* served as a medical and philosophical encyclopedia.

Ibn-Sina defined medicine as "the science by which we learn the various states of the body, in health and when not in health, the means by which health is likely to be lost, and when lost likely to be restored." He also referred to it as an art: "It is the art whereby health is concerned and the art by which it is restored after being lost."

WITCHCRAFT

For a long time in ancient history, witchcraft, magical power and spells were used to antagonize the devil, because people believed he (or it) caused people harm, including sickness and disease. Many cultures believed in witchcraft, including Ancient Egyptians; the Eye of Horus (Figure 10) is a well-known amulet that can be bought at jewelers all over the world. In several cultures it represents "Beyond illuminati" or the third eye, invisible but can see deeply spiritual mental images. In shape it resembles an area located near the center of the brain "Thalamus". In ancient Egypt it was a symbol of responsibility, protection, royal power and good health. On the other hand it is also known as "eye of RA" personifying a powerful destructive force linked with the fierce heat of the sun. Islam, Christianity, and Judaism all refer to magic.

In the Old Testament, witchcraft mostly referred to women who used curses to do harm to others, and Judaism condemned its use and practice. The Jewish word for Sabbath, however, originated from the satanic gathering of witches on that day. In addition, the story of Moses speaks of magic: When he hit the ground with his cane, it turned to a snake that devoured all the other magicians' snakes. In the New Testament, the term "witchcraft" referred mostly to murderers who used poison to kill others, yet Christianity attributes miracles to Jesus, who cured the lepers and gave sight to the blind.

The King James Version of the Bible repeatedly mentions the word or idea of witchcraft, and there are several references to magic, satanic or superstitious events, and whispers of evil spirits.

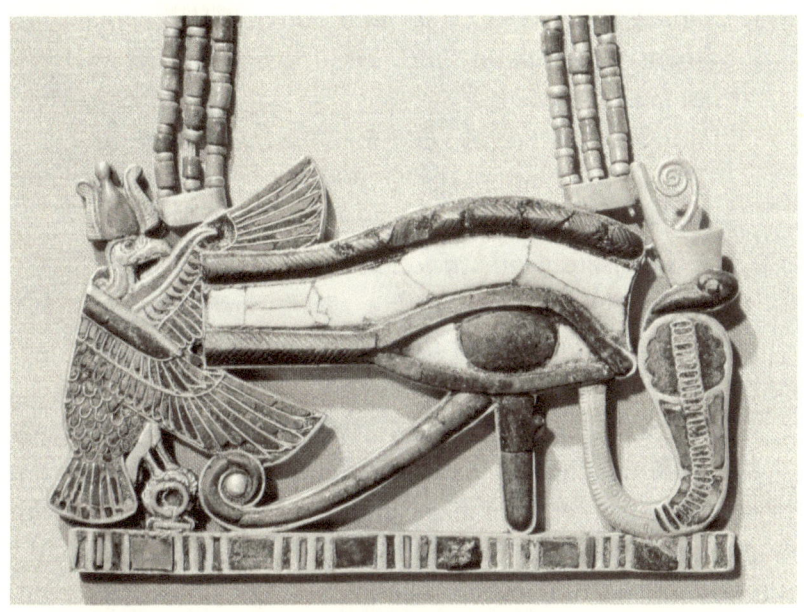

FIGURE 10

Christianity regarded witchcraft as a sin, and sinners had to repent and confess or be forsaken. Examples include the following:

> *And I will cut off witchcrafts out of thine hand; and though shalt have no {more} soothsayers.*
>
> *But there was a certain man called Simon, which beforetime in the same city used sorcery, and bewitched the people of Samaria, giving out that himself was some great one.*
>
> *Now Samuel was dead, and all Israel had lamented him, and buried him in Ramah, even his own city. And Saul had put away those that had familiar spirits and the wizards out of the land.*
>
> *Then said Saul into his servants, seek me a woman that has a familiar spirit, that I may go to her, and*

inquire of her. And his servants said to him, behold, [there is] a woman that hath a familiar spirit in Endor.

Moreover the {works with} familiar spirits, and the wizards, and the images, and the idols, and all the abominations that were spread in the land of Judah and in Jerusalem, did Josiah put away, that might perform the words of the law which were written in the book that Hilkiah the priest found in the house of the Lord.

In the Koran, the holy book of the Moslems, several suras "verses"warn against the use of magic and sorcery. Seeking refuge with God on daybreak from the mischiefs of darkness, "black magic," was recommended. The belief that the devil " jin"can possess someone comes from its mention in the Koran "that God created the angels from light and created the jin from fire." The word "Hasad" meaning envy appeared in the Koran repeatedly. It is about liking something belonging to another person, the evil eye looks at it, and the evil soul follows and pursues it seeking harm to its owner.

The Wiccans, who follow an earth-centered religion, on the other hand do not consider themselves harmful or evil. They believe in nature and consider witchcraft a blessing. Wicca, a modern pagan form of witchcraft was developed in England during the first half of the twentieth century; Gerald Gardner, the author, mathematician, and scriptwriter introduced it to the public in1954. No central authority defines Wicca, but its believers have churches, schools (figure 11), libraries, and teachings based on the philosophy: "If it harm none, do as you will." This religion involves the ritual practice of magic; most of the practitioners believe in duotheism, involving the presence of a god and a goddess symbolized by the moon or mother earth. Others are universal pantheists and believe in a deity that created the cosmos who should be worshiped. They also believe in reincarnation, and the pentagram is their symbol. Gavin and Yvonne Frost founded the Wiccan church and school in the United States in 1968, and they were successful in gaining federal recognition.

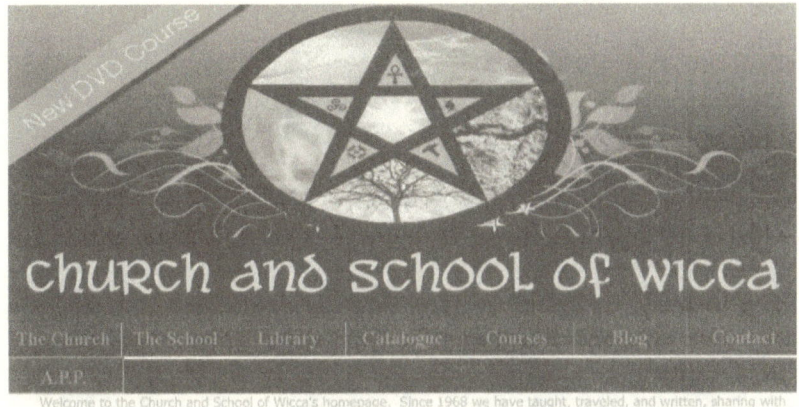

FIGURE 11

The five-pointed star signifies what Wicca believes are the five classical elements: air, fire, water, earth and spirit, which are usually invoked during their magical rituals (figure 12).

These five elements keep you alive and healthy; lacking any one of them is harmful and may cause sickness.

The Wiccans refer to their power as white magic, because they perform it in good faith and good intentions, in contrast to evil black magic. They also claim that their magic simply involves making full use of the five senses and elements. Paul Huson, a British-born author who presently lives in the United States, works extensively in the film and television industry. He wrote several books on witchcraft, including the high-rated *Marketing Witchcraft*. In 1970, he wrote, "The point of magic in witchcraft is to make the bendable world bend to your will. Unless you possess a rock-firm faith in your own powers and in the operability of your spell, you will not achieve the burning intensity of will and imagination which is requisite to make the magic work." In other words, if someone is strong, has faith in his or her powers, and thinks positively, that person can overcome disease.

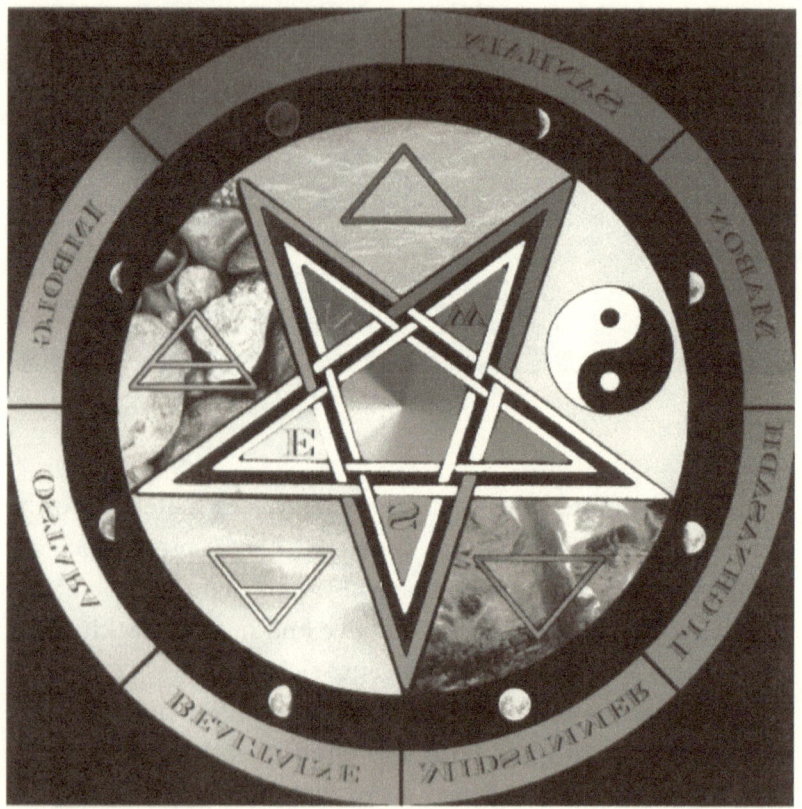

FIGURE 12

Yvonne Frost was kind enough to mail me one of their books titled "A Witch's Guide to Psychic Healing." It mentions homeopathy, soul retrieving, using ones power and other methods of healing.

In medieval Europe, belief in witches was outlawed and considered heresy, particularly at the time of Charlemagne. Toward the end of the Middle Ages, witches, particularly women, were perceived to be in league with the devil and sentenced to death. During the twelfth century, the Inquisition, a decentralized institution within the justice system of the Roman Catholic Church, fought against heretics in many European countries, mainly France. Later, in Germany, Martin Luther—monk, professor of theology, and Protestant reformer—showed no mercy on women who were believed to help the devil; he ordered them to be burned at the stake. Views on these women did not change until the Enlightenment.

In spite of all the religious warnings, there is still a strong belief that evil exists, that magic could counteract it, and that miracles happen. Therefore, the use of holy water in Catholicism and Zamzam water in the Arabian Peninsula are other examples of forces that people believe will repel evil. Believers wash in or drink Zamzam water in the hope that it will cure their particular ailment. For a long time, our mere existence was mind boggling. There are mysteries surrounding childbirth; the process of aging is not fully understood; diseases remain uncontrolled; sudden deaths occur; and plagues wipe out whole communities. In spite of all the research and development in medicine, unknowns are still plentiful today. Out of despair, sick people many times resort to nonmedical means that are a well-accepted tradition in many cultures.

As a child in Egypt, I was scared when the sound of drumbeats far away woke me, and when I asked my parents about the source, they replied, "It is probably a zaar." The zaar ceremony, although nearly vanished now, has been part of the culture since ancient times. It was linked to a belief in witchcraft and was performed as an exorcism ritual, usually for women thought to be inflicted by a spirit causing a chronic incurable illness or a mental condition, or it was done to induce fertility. These ceremonies usually happened in lower-middle-class families under social pressure and stressful obligations; they profit from the zaar psychologically simply from gathering together as in group therapy to vent. The ritual involved loud captivating music (Abu al gheit) to drive away the evil spirit, using a stringed instrument (tanbūra) and drums. Family and friends dance around the suffering person, who joins if she (or he) is able to, not bedridden. The frenzied movements and repeated shaking of the head renders the person anoxic and unconscious, and that is when the spirit leaves the body. A big meal is then served, consisting of unusual and expensive food, sometimes out of season, that the afflicted person ordered. The individual takes advantage of the event and requests dishes he or she desires and could not have gotten under normal circumstances. Although the event has never cured anyone, desperate people continued to practice it for a long time.

The Bride of the Nile by George Ebers describes a yearly festival that takes place in Egypt around the month of August, called Wafaa El-Nil, or fidelity of the Nile. This river is the main water supply and source of life; without it, famine and malnourishment would spread. When the festival started, the Egyptians took the appearance of a particular star as a sign of the Nile waters rising, fertilizing the agricultural land. Too much water caused a disastrous flood, and too little water caused a drought that killed the produce. The story goes that during the festival, the most beautiful virgin would be dressed up like a bride and thrown into the waters of the Nile, so as to eliminate all possibilities of witchcraft from happening. These ceremonies are held to this day, but only as a cultural festive tradition, without the human sacrifice.

The use of amulets, charms, and talismans (*tilasim*) to gain prosperity and happiness and to prevent harm and protect the wearer from evil, danger, misfortune, and disease is also said to originate from ancient Egypt. When you visit countries in the East, many little boutiques sell charms including Cleopatra wheels, seven-point stars, King David's hand, Buddha, the cross, and the *khamsa* (represented by a hand with five fingers, figure 13) ; the latter is believed to defend its wearer from the evil eye. In the Middle Eastern, Indian, and Islamic cultures, the khamsa is said to represent the hand of Fatima, the daughter of Prophet Mohamed, and therefore people believe it prevents or cures sickness. In Judaism, it is also sacred; it is called *hamsa* and represents the hand of Miriam, the sister of Moses. The Turkish Nazar (meaning "sight" in Arabic) is a blue eye-shaped glass or crystal amulet), commonly worn in the Middle East to protect one from the evil eye. I was pleasantly surprised to find out that the evil eye was printed on an Egyptian stamp in commemoration of the fifteenth "Concilium Ophthalmologicum" meeting held in Egypt in 1937. An image of it is present in the foundation of the American Academy of Ophthalmology, "Ophthalmic Heritage and Museum of Vision."

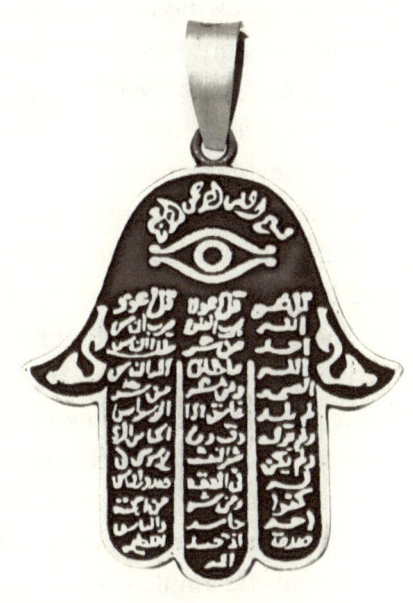

FIGURE 13

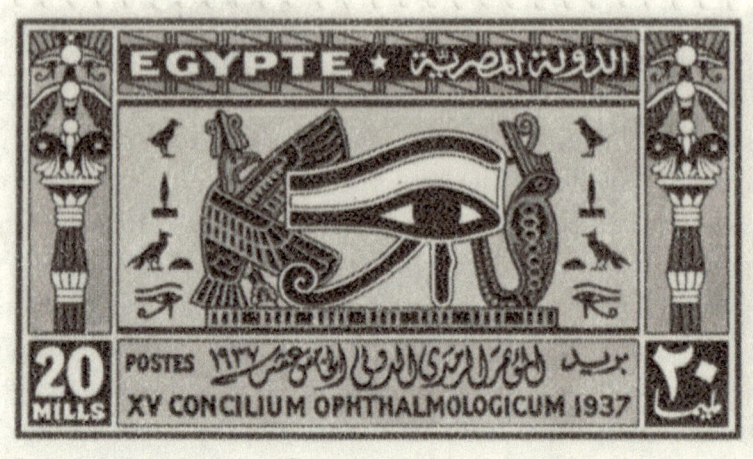

FIGURE 14

My family never believed in witchcraft, a circumstance that made the following story possible. In the mid-1940s, before the discovery of antibiotics, doctors treated infections with bacteriostatics that only stopped bacterial growth like sulpha drugs, rather than bactericidals like antibiotics that kill bacteria; it therefore took a longer time for a patient to develop an immune response to kill the bacteria and be cured. My younger sister was suffering from a bad flu and terrible sore throat. She was out of school for some time, lying in bed. One day, her kindergarten teacher came to see her. She gave my sister a beautiful pendant in the shape of a blue eye, hanging from a golden chain. She told my sister, "Here, wear this; it protects against the evil eye." The five-year-old looked at her, surprised and disappointed, and answered, "But, Miss Fatima, you do not understand. How can this help me? I need something against the evil throat I have. My eye is fine. It does not hurt."

Kabbalistic amulets sold by Gersh Nubirg of Toronto are another example of how people who believe in evil and desperate sick people are led to think that they need personalized amulets, engraved with sacred symbols asking God for his mercy and help, to deal with physical or mental illness. (Kabbalah is the ability to receive help and use positive forces to intensify spiritual influences founded by the Creator.) Philip Berg, the leader of this movement for spiritual connection, guidance, and education and founder of the Kabbalah Center International in the United States was an orthodox rabbi, who died in September 2013. However, the FBI and IRS investigated the center and criticized it as being an opportunistic offshoot of religion.

Blue beads and precious stones like those depicted in ancient Egyptian jewelry, are frequently used for adornments and personal charms to protect someone against illness and misfortune and to save newborns from the evil eye. Archeologists recently recovered blue glass beads from African American sites and consider them to have cultural meaning in West and Central Africa. This brings a question to mind: Was it the protective function of blue that led to the tradition to buy pink clothes for a newborn girl and blue clothes for newborn boys since baby boys were traditionally more desired than girls and therefore needed to be protected from the evil eye?

In the mid-1980s, my husband and I took a trip to Brazil. We went after Christmas and stayed till after the New Year. We had an experience unlike any New Year's Eve celebration we had participated in before. We spent most of the time in Rio de Janeiro, in a five-star hotel in Copacabana, right on the beach. It was fun watching the Brazilian boys play soccer all day on the beach; it was their summer season and a pleasant atmosphere for outdoor partying. The New Year's celebrations started days early, with music and fireworks all along the coast. On New Year's Eve, after midnight, we stood on our balcony, watching an exquisite scene. People dressed in white and carrying lit candles flocked to the beach to jump seven waves and throw flowers into the ocean while making a wish, to bring luck and fortune, because the goddess protecting the sea would make it come true. This tradition is said to come from the mix of African and Indian cultures that developed there over the years. So, no matter how much we advance in education and health, superstition drags the general population into ancient traditions of witchcraft.

Similarly, we still celebrate Halloween in the United States in the twenty-first century. This holiday is thought to have originated with the ancient Celtic festival of *Samhain* ("summer's end"), held to ward off roaming ghosts. In the eighth century, Pope Gregory III designated November 1 as a time to honor all saints and martyrs. It was a celebration of life and death as well as superstition; it was also for people to thank God they survived the previous year through making sacrifices. Shamans attempted to tell fortunes, and the Celtics wore costumes in orange and black to represent fire and death as they danced around a bonfire. The colors and the ghosts from this tradition remain, and the phrase "trick or treat" was introduced to make it more fun.

Shamanism is also mentioned in the *Wellness Dictionary of Minnesota, as part of the Ojibwe Peoples Dictionary, University of Minnesota, historical society of the American Indian studys*; it involves a practitioner reaching an altered state of consciousness to encounter and interact with the spirit world so that he or she can practice divination and healing. Shamans consider themselves messengers between the human world and the world of spirits, and historians believe the practice started from an ancient religion of the Turks and was introduced to the West in 1552. There are many books about shamanism for healing the heart, soul, body, spirit, and mind as well as books for how to practice it. The *Wellness Dictionary of Minnesota* mentions that the ancient Incas made the first recorded use of anesthesia. Shamans got coked up by chewing coca leaves and then drilled holes in the heads of their patients, to let the spirits out, while spitting the chewed substance into the wound to numb the site. This was way before the use of nitrous oxide also called "The Laughing Gas" because of its euphoric effect, for anesthesia, no longer in use, because of its health risks

Most children have watched the movie *The Wizard of Oz* or read the book upon which it's based. This story is but a fantasy about a wicked witch and a wizard who practiced magic. The Harry Potter series includes seven books about Harry's quest to overcome the dark wizard who aims to become immortal and destroy all those who stand in his way. These books were best sellers for children ages five to twelve, and even parents were fascinated with them. Four hundred and fifty million copies have been sold, denoting a high interest in witchcraft. The series was translated into sixty-seven languages. Protestants, Catholics, Orthodox Christians, and some Shiat and Sunni Moslems felt the novels included satanic content and suggested they be taken off the market, but this never happened.

No matter how educated and scientific a country becomes—no matter how much health care advances and how many diseases are eradicated after becoming curable—the signs of fortune tellers and palm readers are still visible on many street corners. After reading the headlines on a newspaper, many people still go to the horoscope column to find out what is waiting for them. Before enjoying the taste of a fortune cookie, many people rush to see what the little paper inside it tells. Therefore, in spite of all the advancements in the medical field, desperately sick people are still told to be positive and fight it out; they resort to prayers, and if that fails, some attempt witchcraft as a last resort.

I keep three valuable books on my coffee table, and I like to share them with my friends who come to visit. The first, *Cézanne*, shows prints of an artist's paintings and provides his biography, including how he became interested in art. The second book is *Life Dream Destinations*, and it has descriptions and photographs of one hundred of the world's best vacations. The third book, my favorite, is *The Power to Heal: Ancient Arts and Modern Medicine*.

It is a photography book of health, healing, and medicine around the world. It contains beautiful photographs depicting traditions and science involved in healing and how it relates to compassion, humanity, and caring. There is a photograph of a New Year's Eve celebration in the Afro-Brazilian religious way, possessed by the goddess Yemoja, with participants praying and hoping for a good fortune and wellness in the following year like we observed on our trip. Another picture depicts the way illness was diagnosed and healed in the South African nation of Swaziland by witchcraft, using seashells, bones, and stones. A picture taken in a Muslim Indian town shows pilgrims from all religions, gathering to visit graves where they all pray for healing; there are other photographs, including a beautiful one of a shrine in France, where people seek cures from different diseases. The book illustrates when science became included in medicine, with pictures of cupping, the art of meditation, the use of herbs, and underwater childbirth; it also demonstrates how the art of healing changed from spiritual, to psychological to scientific.

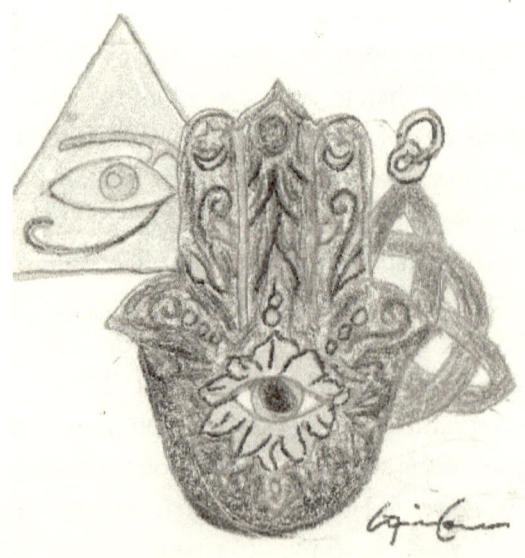

THE AGE OF ENLIGHTENMENT

During the Enlightenment, the art of healing transformed into the science of medicine. This period dominated not only politics, poetry, music, and art but also science and medicine. It followed the dark ages after the fall of the Roman Empire when feudalism hindered upward mobility, wars and famine dominated and bubonic plague devastated the region. The cultural center of thinking transferred from royalty and church to the general public, and the religious basis changed to more realistic reasoning and human emotions. This was when the choral music of Bach and Handel was replaced by the lighter Beethoven and Mozart, and art changed from Baroque to Rococo, as a "witty response to rulers," and the neoclassical. The changes in society embodied the idea of more freedom and a more developed literacy among the bourgeois. The science of medicine excelled in Europe during this age, the late seventeenth through eighteenth century, because of the philosophical, cultural, and intellectual trends at the time. Blind faith, superstition, dogma, and witchcraft were replaced by education, freedom of thought, and stress on logic and reason. Voltaire, the French writer and philosopher (1694–1778), had a big influence on the Enlightenment; he questioned religion and openly criticized the church. The domination of the religious establishment was replaced by free thinkers and writers from the middle class, who changed the study of humanity from the myths of the church to the reality of human existence and rights. Because of these changes, secular intelligence emerged and challenged the clergymen.

When the art of healing changed to involve science intermingled with medicine, things got more complicated. To practice medicine, one had to study more and more as the years passed. Although some knowledge of anatomy began as early as 1600 BCE, as shown in the Edwin Smith surgical papyrus, the human body and all its organs and their relationships needed to be studied more thoroughly. Nomenclature, methods and applications for studying anatomy date back to the Greeks; many medical texts regarding anatomical body parts by various authors were collected in the Hippocratic Corpus. The work of Galen and Avicenna were compiled into modern writings about anatomy, and the first recorded school of anatomy was in Alexandria Egypt from about 300-the second century. Ptolemy who declared himself to be king Ptolemy 1 "Soter" meaning the savior was the first to allow professionals in the medical field to cut and examine dead bodies. It is interesting to know that Leonardo de Vinci was trained in anatomy around 1489 so as to perform his art work, drawing and painting accurately. Other artists from Michelangelo to Rembrandt followed suit. In 1832, Great Britain published *Gray's Anatomy* (figure 15) as a single volume that every medical student since then had to read and study from cover to cover. We did, and our sons did. It is one voluminous book, difficult to carry but easy to study and memorize; it is still present on every medical student's desk, and it accompanies him or her while dissecting a body or studying an organ. Embryology, the study that revealed how a combination of two nonviable cells could gradually develop into a viable human being in the mother's womb or in a test tube, also affected the practice of medicine and the knowledge of human anatomy

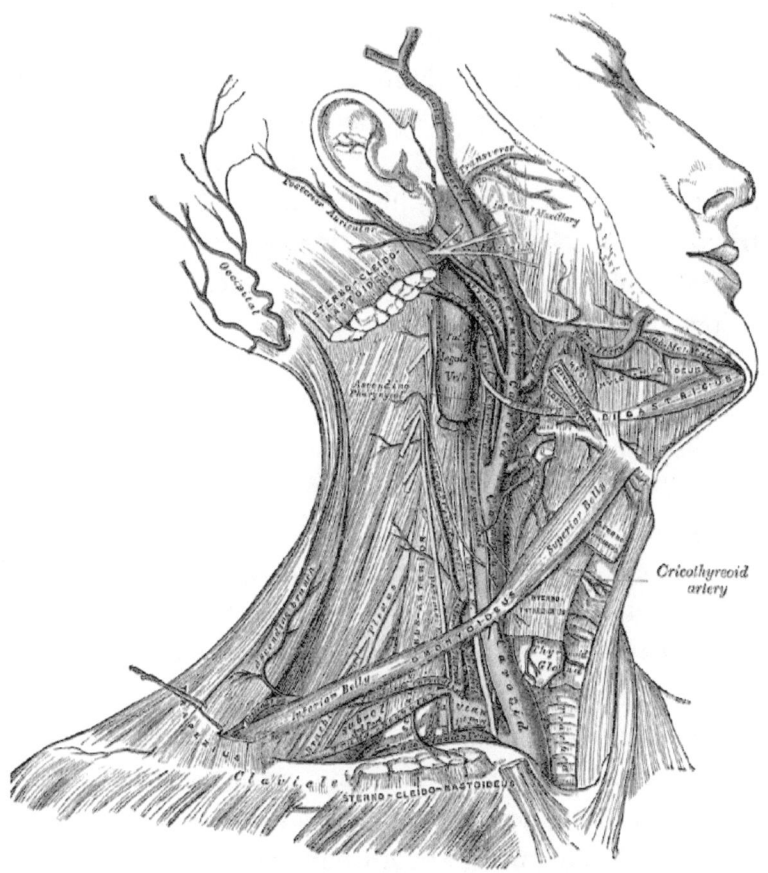

FIGURE 15

Similarly, although Hippocrates understood and wrote about bone structure and function, the science of physiology, which shows how organs work, expanded a great deal during this era. In the mid-1800s, when medicine was equated with science, Rudolf Virchow and Carl Ludwig in Germany as well as Claude Bernard in France gave true birth to physiology; they discovered that functions are achieved by communication between the different body parts in electrical and chemical ways and that the human glands, producing hormones, as well as the nervous system play a major role.

Biology, the study of living creatures, branched into biochemistry, the study of the chemical processes in living organisms, and it revealed how body organs interconnect on the cellular and molecular level. Biochemistry also deals with the structures, functions, and interactions of cellular components, not only the large particles like proteins, carbohydrates, and fats but also interactions on the molecular level. For some time, it was thought that these molecules could only be present in living organisms, (i.e., organic material) research later proved that they could be synthesized in laboratories. Therefore, biochemical advances are what allowed for the discovery of cellular metabolic pathways, DNA, and genes.

"Histology, known earlier as microanatomy, was similarly important to study; it is the branch of biology that deals with various tissues of the body and its microscopic structure. For example, scientists divided the various tissues of the body into: muscular, nervous, connective, and epithelial categories and further divided the epithelial tissue into epithelium, endothelium, and mesothelium, depending upon which part of the body this thin layer of cells covers. Endothelium covers the inner walls of vessels, mesothelium represents the lining of body cavities and protects most internal organs, and epithelium protects the outer body surface and lines the lumen of body organs. Research and advanced knowledge in these branches led to great progress in medical science. Knowledge of how the body functions in health is the first step to knowing how to fight its malfunction in disease.

Although most scientific developments in medicine were a product of research, some major ones resulted from a lucky moment. Louis Pasteur, born in France (1822–1895), discovered that alcohol soured because of microorganisms called bacteria. They caused fermentation, and they could be destroyed by heating beverages to certain temperatures and then quickly cooling. This process was named pasteurization after this scientist, and since that time pasteurized milk is devoid of disease-causing bacteria, and humans can drink it without boiling it. Before this discovery, boiling milk killed bacteria, but it also killed vitamins and destroyed the structure of proteins. Pasteur, who grew bacteria for experiments in culture media, accidentally exposed a chicken to an attenuated (weak) strain of a bacterial culture and discovered that the fowl became resistant to the cultured organism; this incident gave him the idea of vaccination. He experimented by exposing healthy people to weak cultures of bacteria, so that they would develop resistance. He thereby created vaccines for anthrax, rabies, and cholera in addition to smallpox. He was called father of microbiology, and the Pasteur Institute was opened in 1888 to honor him.

Robert Koch, a German physician (1843–1910) is also considered a founder of modern bacteriology. Building on Pasteur's work, he discovered Bacillus anthracis, the causative organism of Anthrax, and worked on ways to identify other bacteria under the microscope. He also developed chemicals to attack specific disease-causing bacteria, tuberculosis in 1882 and cholera in 1883. Since that time, microbiology—the science of small life—led to great progress in medicine. It allowed scientists to view these minute creatures that caused disease, and many times epidemics, with microscopes. The organisms were cultured, grown on appropriate media, and used either in combination with the appropriate medication or to develop a preventative vaccine. However, bacteria have the ability to mutate, so we keep discovering new ones, which can also develop resistance to medication used against them. It is an ongoing challenge to find new means to combat them. I read an article in the General Surgery News about hospital battles with superbugs. It describes how hospitals, pharmacies, and the CDC (centers for disease control and prevention) are trying to combat a hospital-based infection where the causative bacterium, Klebsiella pneumonia, is becoming resistant to antibiotics that were successfully used against it before; in fact, it caused an epidemic in one institute with a 40 percent mortality rate for those infected. Similar incidences were reported in other hospitals necessitating the development of infection control committees to combat and implement preventive measures against "nosocomial" hospital acquired infections.

It is obvious that all these bacteria would not have been identified without the use of the microscope. Therefore, the invention of the microscope was one of the greatest scientific discoveries during Europe's revival from the Dark Ages. Without it, no microbiologist, histologist, or pathologist could have done his or her job. It took several stages for this instrument to reach its final shape and usage; in fact, at the beginning, it was not used for medicine at all. A glass manufacturer discovered that a biconcave lens enlarged objects and used it as a magnifying glass; this type of lens was reshaped to be used for spectacles till around the year 1590. Further experiments were run with several such lenses set in elongated tubes, and they kept enlarging objects to increasing degrees. As children, we played with lenses we let sun rays pass through a biconvex lens, placed a sheet of paper underneath at a certain distance until it burned, and we learned that the distance was the focal length of that lens.

The true father of microscopy, Anton Van Leeuwenhoek, built his own instruments reaching magnifications that allowed him to see and describe tiny living organisms in a drop of water, and he called them bacteria. The improved light microscope can only detect objects that are equal to or larger than half the wavelength of light—that is, 0.275 micrometers. Therefore, viruses we used to refer to as organisms not detected by the light microscope, could only be visualized and studied after the year 1930, when the electron microscope was invented. Electrons are sped up in a vacuum until their wavelength is as short as one hundred thousandth of white light, enabling the detection of smaller objects. I was privileged to work on one of the earliest electron microscopes during my fellowship in Houston, Texas, in 1964. I was so elated to see the causative organisms of disease I never could before and to observe how they multiplied and affected the cells they attacked and the mechanism by which they led to their destruction.

Each year, more scientific work was introduced into the medical field. Edward Jenner (1749–1823) became known as the father of immunology because he noticed that milkmaids who caught the cowpox "vaccinia" virus from the cows they were milking did not catch a smallpox infection, which was a deadly disease at the time. Since his discovery, smallpox has been completely eradicated. Smallpox "variola" scars appear on the faces of mummies from the eighteenth through twentieth Egyptian dynasties, and the virus was supposedly brought from Egypt to India and later to the West, causing large-scale epidemics. It used to be well known that one could induce immunity against smallpox by inoculation or insufflation of infectious material, such as scabs from the skin lesions of a sick person, blown into the nose of a healthy person; it would cause him or her to develop a mild form of the disease and immunity to the severe deadly form. This process, called variolation, led the aforementioned Edward Jenner, a British physician in the eighteenth century, to develop the first successful vaccine against smallpox; scientifically controlled vaccination has since replaced the haphazard procedure of insufflations, and it became a widespread protective method all over the world. The term vaccination was derived from the Latin word "vaca," meaning "cow." The practice of vaccination saved the world; it was a successful response to the deadly epidemic that hastened the decline of the Roman Empire, killing seven million people.

Wilhelm Conrad Roentgen (1845–1923) exemplifies that science in fields other than medicine had a gigantic effect on the progress of diagnostics in medical science. He was a mechanical engineer and professor of physics. Around 1895, while conducting an experiment with vacuum tubes containing electrodes, he noticed a glow and thought it was caused by a mysterious ray, and so he named it an x-ray. The emitted rays could be reflected, and they appeared on photographic plates. Continuing these experiments, Roentgen could get pictures of radio-opaque objects. He was awarded the Nobel Prize in physics in 1901, and his invention became a very important diagnostic tool in medicine. Heart and lung disease were clarified; bone fractures and tumors could be visualized; and gallbladder and kidney stones could be identified.

In addition to the progress of diagnostic tools in medicine, there were also improvements in preventive measures during this period of time, including quarantine, isolation, and vaccination; most importantly, diseases were combatted and cured with the use of drugs. Many medicines were initially discovered by accident and later needed to be purified and artificially synthesized. Theophylline, for example, an effective treatment for asthma and COPD (Chronic Obstructive Pulmonary Disease), was originally discovered as an extract from tea leaves, and it is now synthesized and chemically developed. The story goes that a man was relaxing in the shade under a tree, and when a leaf fell into his drink, he continued drinking and found himself more alert and stimulated, for it raises the blood pressure, stimulates the nervous system and increases the heart beat. With further experimentation, theophylline was proven to be a potent diuretic as well.

In 1884, Sigmund Freud, then a young physician in Vienna, wrote about cocaine derived from coca leaves. He noticed that natives in South America had been chewing the leaves for centuries to alleviate pain. Similarly, quinine—extracted from the bark of the cinchona tree in Peru—was discovered first as a muscle relaxant, and then it became the most successful medicine in treating Malaria; its synthetic relative, quinidine, has been effectively used in heart conditions for a long time. In fact, the first known heart medicine was discovered accidentally in an English garden in 1799, when a physician noted the effect of dried leaves of the common foxglove plant, Digitalis purpurea, (figure 16) on cardiac ailment. The foxglove family of plants is native to western and southwestern Europe, western and central Asia, Australia, and northwestern Africa. It is grown as an ornamental plant because of its vivid flowers, ranging in color from various purples to shades of grey to pure white; they are very pretty but dangerous. In fact, they are the most poisonous plants grown in gardens and have many times been fatal when ingested; mere contact with the leaves may cause diarrhea, nausea, and vomiting, but the active ingredient, digi-

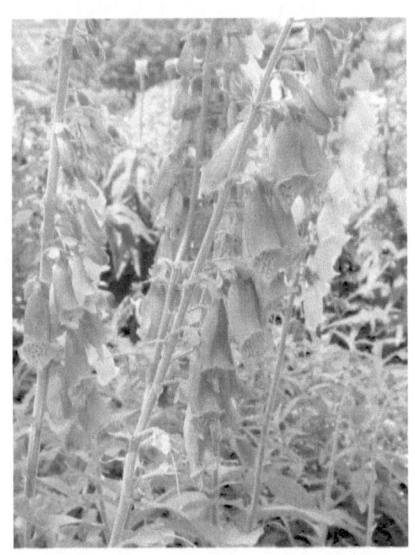

FIGURE 16

talis, has helped in treating many aspects of heart disease, ranging from regulating pulse rate to cardiac failure, for hundreds of years.

In 1910, a German bacteriologist formulated an arsenic compound that was the only effective treatment for syphilis for a long time. In the early 1920s, Gerhard Domagk was experimenting with dyes at I. G. Farben, one of the largest dye companies at the time. While working with an orange-red dye called prontosil, he produced a sulfa antimicrobial bacteriostatic drug that stops bacterial growth. It was used to ameliorate infections till the time when the bactericidal penicillin that kills bacteria was discovered.

In 1928, Sir Alexander Fleming of Scotland (1881–1955) made an accidental discovery that had a major effect in saving lives. While he was working in a hospital laboratory, a plate with a culture of staph bacteria was accidentally contaminated by a blue-green mold. At the site of contamination, the bacterial colonies disappeared. He realized that these bacteria had died, so he grew the mold in a pure culture and discovered that it produced a substance that killed bacteria that caused a number of infections and diseases. Although it took till the early 1940s to develop this product in a purified form that could be used in medicine, this was a true revolution: the birth of penicillin. This turning point led to the production of numerous antibiotics that were more effective and had a wider use of applications than previous ones. It is said that ancient Egyptians used rotten food with mold to heal infected wounds not knowing the mode of action.

Aspirin, the wonder drug that made the German company Bayer so famous, was introduced in its (Bayer Cross on The Wall) trademarked form (figure 17) in the year 1899, after Felix Hoffman, a chemist, formulated it. The cross is not the Bayer trademark in the USA anymore, though it is in other countries, yet is still hanging shining on the Bayer healthcare's building in Whippany, New Jersey (Figure 18). Hippocrates, the father of modern medicine (460 BC–377 BC), made use of the active ingredient in aspirin; he treated fever, headache, and other pains using a powder made from the bark and leaves of the Willow

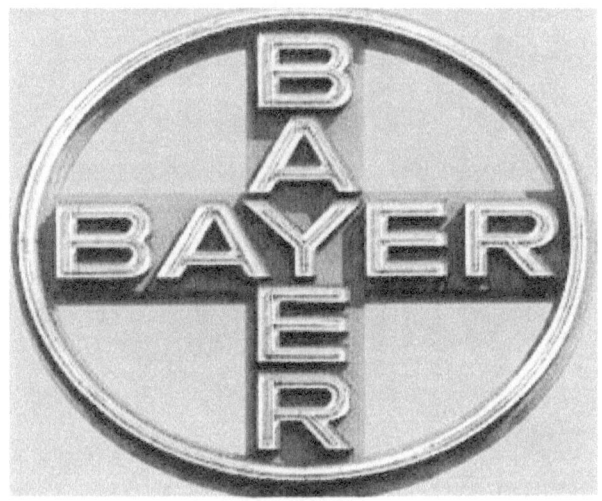

FIGURE 17

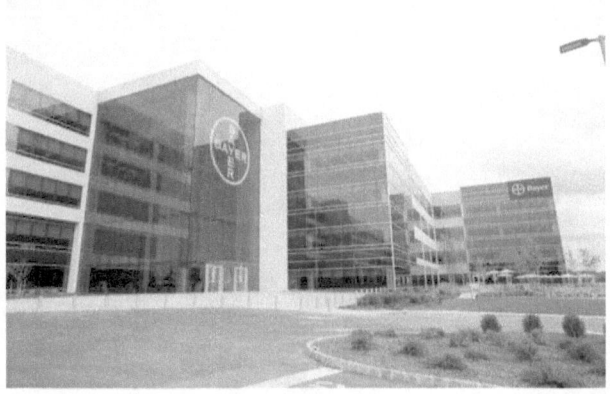

FIGURE 18

Salix tree (figure 19), and its flower clusters "Catkin" (Figure 20) of the genus *Salix*. It contained salicin, from which salicylic acid, the active ingredient in aspirin, was developed. So, pharmacology—the study and usage of drugs—initially arose from accidental discoveries and substances found in nature, mainly plants, but, over time, it changed to include analytical scientific

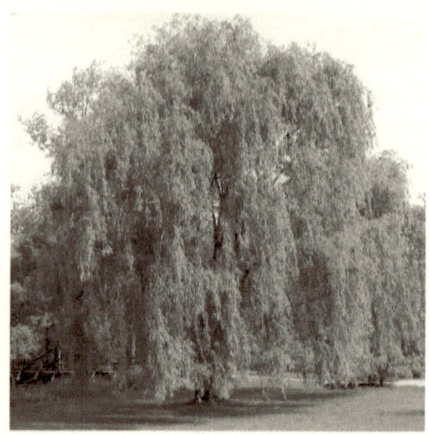

FIGURE 19

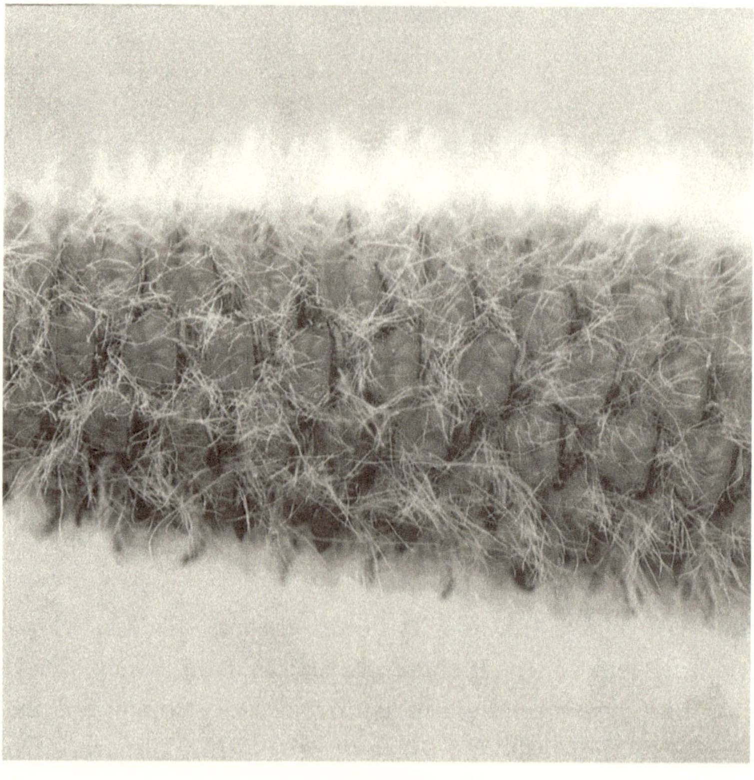

FIGURE 20

procedures and strict regulations by the FDA (Food and Drug Administration) and interaction between the European and US pharmacopeia. During the period of scientific enlightenment, many plants that were accidentally found to have medicinal effects were purified to extract their active ingredients; later, many of these ingredients could be chemically produced and manufactured into pills.

The basic science of pharmacology, which started around 1828, deals not only with discovering a given drug but also with screening it for desired activity, determining the way it functions, observing which organ or organism it acts upon— up to the cellular level, and discovering the proper dosage and whether there are any toxic or undesirable side effects. These tests are done in vitro (in test tubes and culture plates) or in vivo (with live animals, mice, rats, guinea pigs, or dogs) and then on humans. I can still recall our practical lab sessions in medical school in physiology and pharmacology; they were a lot of fun. It was a well-known fact that an isolated organ or tissue that had been freshly removed from the body remained functional for several hours, in a bath containing a solution of saline through which oxygen was bubbled. We performed experiments on isolated hearts, strips of skeletal muscle, and stomachs from frogs and rabbits; these were suspended so that their contractions and relaxation was transmitted to a stylet that would write on a rotating drum covered with blackened paper. This kymograph recorded motions or pressure graphically. It allowed us to see the effect of different drugs, we manually added to the solutions where the organs we were testing had been placed.

One of the most informative studies for the potency of a medicine, the double-blind study, uses experimental and control groups of human beings to test the effectiveness of a drug.

Neither the subject nor the investigator knows whether he or she is using the drug or a placebo "fake none-effective product". The idea is to exclude any psychological prejudgment of the result. After the treatment is given and the results and the effects are tabulated, it is decoded and announced what each participant received, and the medicine is deemed to be effective if it performed differently than the placebo.

It saddens me when I think back to the times in our residency when we were asked to participate in experimentation with new drugs. Representatives of big pharmaceutical companies like Ciba, Merck, Sandoz, and others would provide our professors with newly developed medicines, which they suggested we prescribe for patients complaining of specific symptoms or known to have a certain kind of disease. We had to test the drugs' effectiveness and determine whether they produced any side effects or complications. These were considered research projects; the results were published in medical journals and compared with medicines already in use. Publishing papers is a must in universities and is needed to secure promotions. No one asked patients for their consent in these medical trials, and the drugs were not yet approved for marketing, so people in third-world countries were used for blind human studies only after the drugs were proven to be effective in guinea pigs. In retrospect, I realized that our patients were unknowingly used for testing new drugs at just one level higher than guinea pigs. So, we and our patients actively participated for some time in these double-blind studies.

When my parents were practicing medicine and when my peers and I started, medical practice was limited in spite of all the new scientific developments. Medicine was practiced the old-fashioned way. Many doctors had offices downtown, and patients selected whom to visit by word of mouth. There was a deep feeling of trust and compassion. Some just visited a neighborhood physician; it did not make much difference to them. Frequently, a patient did not even go to a doctor's office, but instead the doctor would make house calls to the patient who was lying comfortably in his or her bed at home. A doctor could make several house calls on a single day, carrying a bag with such supplies as a mercury thermometer dipped in alcohol, a stethoscope, a sphygmomanometer (blood-pressure machine), a pack of antiseptics, commonly used medications, and his prescription pad. The patient would be in bed, surrounded by a loving family till the doctor arrived. It was customary to offer the physician a cup of coffee before going to the patient's room. After seeing the patient, the doctor was handed a bar of soap (for hand washing), offered a spray of eau de cologne, given a clean ironed towel, and invited to the living room to discuss the case and mode of treatment with the family. At the end of the conversation, someone handed the physician an envelope containing his fees; it would go directly into his pocket, no questions asked. The family decided on the customary fee, depending on how much they appreciated the doctor's effort and advice. Patients were rarely sent to a lab for tests or to the hospital. It was not uncommon for a doctor to examine a patient for free, as a courtesy, if the family might not be able to afford the fees. Frequently, a doctor would be rewarded specially in small towns or villages with a big basket of fruit, live chicken or other poultry, or homemade pastry and cookies instead of or in addition to a fee in cash.

Scientific advances in medicine keep growing year after year, and while we were practicing, we had to learn about new developments by attending yearly courses for continuing medical education. Changes were happening at a very fast pace, and the practice of medicine expanded. Patients who had shunned hospitals accepted the fact that they needed to be admitted to receive better care and observation. Patients who were scared of having blood drawn agreed to the fact that laboratory tests had to be performed for a proper diagnosis and treatment. They also realized that more diseases had become curable, and they should not give up easily; rather, they should keep fighting for their lives and try new medications and procedures.

When the new scientific knowledge became too overwhelming for any one person to absorb, retain, and practice, doctors began to specialize in a particular area. We heard about cardiologists, who focused on knowledge about diseases of the heart; pulmonists, specializing in diseases of the lungs; gastroenterologists, mainly concerned with the stomach, intestines, and colon; hepatologists, who knew the most about liver diseases; and hematologists, who investigated blood diseases. We also got endocrinologists; immunologists; rheumatologists; nephrologists, for kidneys; neurologists, involved with the nervous system; orthopedists, mending bones and joints; and so on. Every organ or system in the body soon had its own specialist, and the general practitioner's office became primarily a referring station. The compassionate, trustworthy, and private patient-doctor relationship went out the window.

When my classmates and I graduated from medical school, according to the British system, the certificate read, "MB BCH," which stood for a bachelor's degree in medicine and chirurgie (surgery). The University of Glasgow, Oxford, Cambridge, Liverpool, and Edinburgh all used this terminology. The initials after our names later became MD, medical doctor, comparable to the highest degrees in other sciences, PhD, or doctor of philosophy, indicating general knowledge of all fields of medicine. Now doctors are named according to their specialty.

In the sixteenth century in Great Britain, the barber-surgeon was a skilled common practitioner charged with looking after soldiers and providing medical assistance to the wealthy; they provided a variety of tasks like extracting teeth, cutting off hangnails, removing gallstones, setting fractures, treating abscesses, performing bloodletting, and other minor surgeries. Under pressure from the medical profession in 1745, surgeons split from barbers. In 1800, The Royal College of Surgeons came into being, and surgeons applied to become fellows there. Because of this history, the degree awarded to surgeons for the longest time was M CH or MS. And for traditional reasons, holders of the FRCS (Fellow of the Royal College of Surgeons) kept their title as master or mister rather than doctor. Surgeons were trained through an apprenticeship, at the end of which they were examined and given a diploma, while physicians after the Middle Ages had to hold a university degree. Of course, at present, every physician and surgeon has to hold a university degree and have sufficient training to allow board certification in his or her specialty. The medical field has expanded to also include nurses and nursing aids, technicians and technologists in laboratories and radiology, secretaries, specialists in medical records, nutritionists, dietitians, psychologists and psychiatrists, physical therapists, pharmacists, and many more. This causes confusion for the patient, who may be referred from one specialty to the other in search of better care.

Anesthesiology was not developed till the late 1800s. Early on, an assistant to the surgeon would physically hold or strap down patients undergoing minor procedures; in later centuries, the patient would drink alcohol or inhale nitrous oxide known as laughing gas. Ether was used in 1846 and then chloroform in 1847; many times, these substances were toxic for the patient and were therefore called "the choking gases." The nurse had to literally wrestle the patients during preparation for surgery, so surgery was considered to be a brutal business. As mentioned before, Sigmund Freud suggested the use of cocaine as a local anesthetic to alleviate pain by acting on the peripheral sensory nerve endings. Controlling airways during anesthesia and preventing the patient from choking by use of an endo-tracheal air tube was only introduced in 1920; intravenous induction, a method wherein the patient falls asleep before any other measures are taken, was introduced in 1930; and the use of muscle relaxants was started in the 1940s. These measures and sedation rendered anesthesia more tolerable and minimally dangerous.

Pathology, both clinical and anatomical, the science of differentiating between normal and diseased tissues and body fluids, assisted physicians markedly. It helped diagnostically, lab test results confirm or disprove clinical diagnoses, and educationally, by providing more information about the results of their work. Many times, physicians wait for a word from a pathologist to tell them what went wrong and how to treat it. After surgery, when the patient asks his or her surgeon what the doctor found, the surgeon would answer, "Let us wait for the pathology report to discuss a final diagnosis." Pathologists themselves learn a lot from their research. For example, performing autopsies may reveal the hidden facts of what happened in a patient's body and whether the previous diagnosis was accurate. There is a saying, "He who laughs last, laughs best." I would add, "He who finds out last, knows best." The pathologist is usually that person. Since my retirement in 1997 and because of the rapid expansion in medical science, not to mention the tremendous improvements in diagnostics and treating procedures, I try to keep up with what is new in the general field of medicine particularly my specialty by keeping in contact with and staying as a member of the College of American Pathologists. I receive their magazines and read their journals. In these periodicals, I read about current research and developments, recent techniques and procedures I was not aware of during my practice, new tests and applications I never trained for, and other unbelievable advancements in such a short time. It makes me wonder what is coming next, and I fully agree with my granddaughter who once said, "I can't wait to see how technology will develop in the next few years."

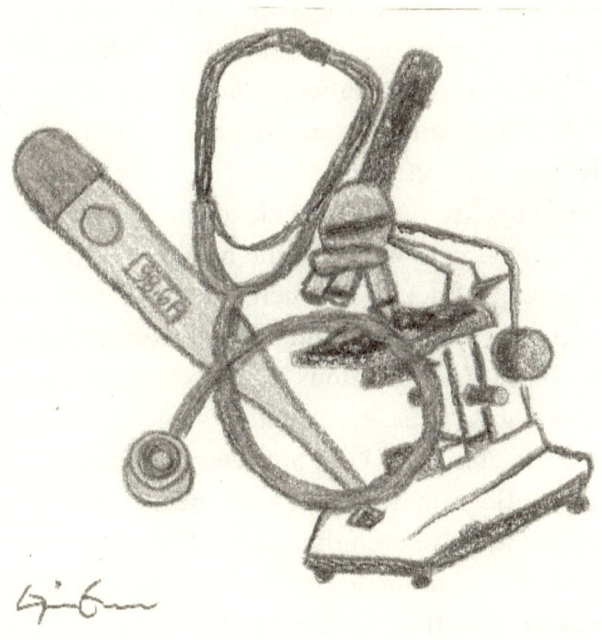

INTRODUCTION OF TECHNOLOGY

I do not intend to go as far back as the year 1816, when Rene Laennec invented the stethoscope. At the time, it was a great help for doctors; before its invention, doctors had to lean down and stick their ears to the patient's chest to listen to heart beats, respiratory movements or any deviation from the normal. Similarly, I am not referring to the invention of the primitive ophthalmoscope to view the back of the eye in 1851, the laryngoscope in 1855 to examine the back of the throat and the upper respiratory tract, or the mercury sphygmomanometer in 1896, which is now obsolete and banned from being sold to the public because of its hazardous mercury content and has been replaced by digital ones, even though some of them are not as accurate or reliable. And I am not referring to the invention of the electrocardiogram in 1901 or even the introduction of adhesive bandages in 1920, even though the latter was considered to be a marvelous invention, for it assisted in rapid wound healing and prevented infection. I am not even referring to other milestones in medical technology like the electroencephalogram, which records brain waves, allowing the evaluation of changes in the brain functions and enabling a German physiologist to reveal brain activity during sleep in 1924. My focus is not on the invention of the iron lung, the ventilator that regulated negative and positive pressures for artificial respiration in 1927, or renal dialyzers in 1945 that allowed a kidney transplant patient to survive and live longer than one year; at the time, it was considered to be a big success.

Instead of all these medical technologies, I wish to discuss the great paradigm shift that started in the second half of the twentieth century, continuing rapidly to the present time. During this time, the practice of medicine changed from a one-on-one relationship between the patient and physician and expanded into a complex medical field because of the massive addition of new technology. Medicine had formerly depended on the (art of healing), doctor's observational and interpretational skills, treating the patient accordingly, but it became increasingly dependent on diagnostic technology and advanced curative methods.

This was also the period of time when the field of medicine included several alliances and paramedical personnel. New diagnostic technology required laboratories with specialized technologists and technicians as well as microbiologists and biochemists and needed to be equipped with new machinery and updated diagnostic tools; x-ray departments needed general radiologists, interventional radiologists and radiotherapists. In addition, new methods of treatment developed new products year after year, and this required pharmaceuticals and pharmacies to expand. Nurses and nursing aids needed more training and experience to keep up with new developments in charting patient's medical information and keeping electronic records. In addition, institutions specializing in pain therapy; physical therapy; general, cardiac, and pulmonary rehab; and social services developed and expanded services.

Because of the tremendous increase in technological innovations and the tremendous expansion in medical technological procedures, doctors started to subspecialize, so general medical practice branched into even more branches. For example, cardiologists, who take care of heart conditions, divided themselves into noninvasive and invasive specialists. In the latter group some introduce coronary balloons and stents; others only deal with pacemakers and defibrillators to treat irregular heartbeats.

Pulmonologists also became noninvasive, examining and treating lung diseases, and invasive, using endoscopic techniques and bronchoscope tools; gastroenterologists who research symptoms of dyspepsia, stomach and intestinal ailments are now trained to perform upper and lower endoscopies and endoscopic retrograde cholangiopancreatographies. Orthopedists restricted themselves to only feet, knees, hips, spines, or hands; urologists, who provide cystoscopic investigative and curative procedures, also specialized in their own fields.

Patients have become so fascinated with the expansion in technology and its effectiveness in early diagnosis and better patient care and treatment, that they often have better confidence in technology than in the doctor's clinical skills and judgment; they request technological investigative procedures even when the doctor does not recommend them. Doctors are also realizing that by using available technology, many hidden medical conditions can be discovered early enough for them to be completely curable. Therefore, the practice of examining a sick patient shifted from seeing the patient and then ordering tests based on the diagnosis or suspected condition to the present practice of ordering an array of tests and scans before the patient walks into the Doctor's office. The traditional practice of looking at body parts from the outside changed to examining various body parts and tissues from the inside out, with the introduction of laparoscopy and endoscopy.

An interesting article related to this new technology was published in the June 29, 1997, edition of the *New York Times*. Lawrence K. Altman wrote a piece titled "The Inside Story" about a history of noninvasive medical introspection. This article mentioned a book by Bettyann Holtzmann Kevles, *Naked to the Bone: Medical Imaging in the Twentieth Century*. In her book, she referred to the shooting of President James A. Garfield in 1881 and how doctors failed to locate the bullet that ultimately led to his demise. At the time, Alexander Graham Bell, famous for the invention of the telephone, tried to help by using his sound theory to locate the bullet. (Bell's idea behind his invention was to convert sound waves into electrical signals and vice versa.) He passed an exploring coil over the president's body, assuming that it would signal the location of the bullet if an electronic field could be generated and that way it could be easily extracted. His idea was to use sound in diagnostics, similar to the use of the stethoscope, although he was well aware that the stethoscope was only a sound amplifier, but his trial did not work, and he failed to locate the bullet. An x-ray would have solved this mystery and saved the president's life, but it was not implemented in medical use until over a decade later.

It is common knowledge that the Bell Telephone Company, organized in Boston, Massachusetts, in the mid-1880s, provided communication services to most of the United States and Canada during that time. Bell Labs later moved to New York and New Jersey for better tax benefits; in 1984, it evolved into the American Telephone and Telegraph Company, AT&T, and made noteworthy developments. However, the acoustic era really started long before that, in the year 1877, when Thomas Edison successfully recorded sound on tinfoil wrapped around a rotating cylinder; he patented the phonograph with its loudspeaker. I was pleasantly surprised to read that the song he recorded for his gramophone was, "Mary had a little lamb." We still sing it to our children and grand children not realizing how much the Bell Company contributed to the progress in the medical field.

The paradigm shift in medicine was not the use of sound, but came from implementing ultrasound technology. Ultrasound is the energy produced by sound waves twenty thousand or more vibrations per second, far above the frequency of sound the human ear can hear. Lazzaro Spallanzani first experimented with bats in 1790, but it wasn't till 1794 that there was evidence to demonstrate that bats navigated by sound inaudible to humans, not vision. The same was found to be true about mice, cats, dogs, and dolphins; in fact, that is why these creatures feel earthquakes long before humans do; they are sensitive to ultrasound. In 1880, Jack and Pierre Curie generated and detected ultrasonic waves in air and water, and Pierre Curie discovered the connection between electrical voltage energy and pressure on certain quartz crystal material, called the piezoelectric effect. The theory is that there is an accumulated electric charge in certain solid materials—notably, crystals and ceramics. Curiously enough, this type of charge was also found in human bone and in minute particles like DNA and proteins. This electricity can be generated by applying certain pressure, and the process can be reversed to produce ultrasonic waves. Spontaneous polarization of crystals takes place due to the separate accumulation of the positive and negative charges in the material. When pressure or stress is applied, the charges shift, and the size of the electrical charge produced depends on the elasticity of the target; thus, the reflected signal is also a function of this elasticity, enabling mapping of the organ under investigation. Pierre Curie applied this principal to invent what he called the transducer. The instrument gave off focused, high-frequency ultrasound waves that were reflected back to the transducer when applied to organs and tissues inside the human body, allowing pictures to appear on a screen.

The contribution of ultrasound technology, also called sonography, to medical diagnostics was tremendous. However, conventional ultrasound imaging got its true start in the late 1930s, when Doctor Karl Dussik implemented it in diagnosing brain tumors. His study involved the use of the transducer, ultrasound gel, and a scanner to expose the body to high-frequency sound waves, show the structure or movements in the organs, and display the images on the scanner in thin flat sections of the body. This method was mainly used in gynecological evaluations, and it was later adapted to produce three-dimensional images. Ultrasound tests can identify appendicitis, gallstones, intra-abdominal and chest tumors, fractures, and many other conditions. Later, Doppler measurements were used in sonography (a change in wave frequency) to examine blood flow in arteries. Later still, the technology was developed to be used in obtaining ultrasound-guided biopsies like from lungs and breasts without requiring an open incision. In 1953, Inge Edler in Lund, Sweden, used ultrasound to obtain well-defined echoes moving synchronously with the heartbeats (an echocardiogram), and by 1955, he could use it to diagnose mitral valve stenosis that is narrowing of the opening between the left upper and lower chambers of the heart. This was a great advancement for cardiac patients. The Vscan is the latest in ultrasound technology. It is a pocket-sized high-resolution ultrasound device that the doctor can carry around like a stethoscope, use to examine a patient, read the echogram, and discuss it with the patient on the spot, without delay.

Endoscopy was another great contribution to modern medical diagnostics. It is not completely noninvasive, but it led to the use of minimally invasive procedures to replace open surgery. It also changed the mode of examining patients from the old method: inspection (viewing), palpation (feeling), percussion (tapping), and auscultation (listening)—the way my peers and I were taught—to the new idea of introspection, or looking at the internal story. The latter entails examining hollow body organs from their inside. Scopes have been used more and more frequently since the first model was developed in 1806 in Mainz, Germany. Philipp Bozzini, a medical doctor, produced a very primitive one called a *Lichtleiter*, or light conductor, to visualize and inspect the ear, mouth, nose, cervix, and rectum from the inside. It consisted of a tube speculum, mirrors, and artificial candlelight. It was later modified, and in 1853, a brighter turpentine light source and the addition of lenses to the mirror improved visualization; Gustave Trouve developed the first electrically illuminated scope in 1869. Rigid endoscopes were manufactured en masse, starting in 1906; they were of limited usage, and in 1911, Sussmann developed the advanced flexible gastroscope, illuminated by miniature electric lamps that reflected light from external sources. The best innovation in endoscopes was the fiber-optic model invented by Fernando Alves Martins of Portugal in 1963. It simplified the procedure and improved visualization of lesions like ulcers, polyps, bleeding points, and small tumors in areas that were out of sight before. This instrument is designed to have great flexibility; it consists of bundles of flexible glass fibers able to transmit the required image to the screen or to be photographed by a microcamera; the light source is channeled to the tip of the instrument.

During the early 1980s, many of our colleagues in surgery took a few days off work to train for a new technology. They took intensive courses in laparoscopy; at the time, it was mainly laparoscopic cholecystectomy. The important part of training was in eye-hand coordination, because the procedure differed from the conventional surgery. Conventionally, the surgeon saw the structures in the abdominal cavity through a wide open incision in the abdominal wall; after separating the abdominal wall flaps by the use of retractors, the surgeon took out the gallbladder under direct supervision. In the new procedure, the internal abdominal structures are visualized through a keyhole opening in the abdominal wall, via images displayed on a TV screen. The surgeon works on the abdominal cavity, introducing instruments through another hole while watching the procedure on the monitor.

Before the introduction of laparoscopy, one sometimes heard the patient ask the surgeon before going into the operating room, "Doctor, what do you think—is it serious? Is there hope?" The surgeon would answer, "It will depend on our findings. We need to open and see. We need to do an exploratory laparotomy." That procedure meant opening the abdomen through a wide incision and looking around the area to assess the extent of the disease, determine what could be done next according to the situation, and decide what needed to be taken out. After going through all this trouble, the surgeon sometimes had bad news and would have to face the anxious patient and his or her family to tell them that all he did was open and close. The disease was too advanced and widespread, and nothing could be removed during surgery. Thanks to laparoscopy, this does not happen routinely anymore, and exploratory laparotomies have vanished completely, replaced by laparoscopic exploration. The laparoscopic approach serves the patient by providing early diagnosis, less invasive procedures, shorter duration of surgery, less exposure to anesthesia, less pain, speedier recovery, and much shorter hospitalization. In fact, many times this procedure can be performed on an outpatient basis.

Experimenting with laparoscopy started in Germany in the early 1900s on animals. The procedures were refined and popularized over the years, but they were not in vogue for surgeons until the right instrumentation was invented and computer-chip television cameras were developed. Gynecologists performed the first laparoscopic salpingectomy in 1976, and then a surgeon performed the first appendectomy using laparoscopy in 1981. Since those surgeries, more and more laparoscopic diagnostic and curative procedures have been performed, and increasingly larger organs and masses can be removed, such as the stomach, colon, and even kidney with minimal invasion or destruction of body tissue.

Since the early 1970s, computerized imaging also became an important diagnostic tool in medicine. Its sensitivity and early diagnostic capability make it strongly indicated in preventive medicine; the earlier the identification of a tumor, the higher the possibility of its eradication and cure. Computed tomography (CT), or computerized axial tomography (CAT scan), uses a series of x-ray views from different angles and serial cross-sectional images of an organ through perpendicular and transverse axes to the smallest size possible. This way, doctors can identify tumors measured in millimeters before they grow to a more obvious size. Tomography was experimented with at UCLA as early as 1959, but the first reliable commercial CT scanner was invented in 1967. There is an amazing story of how this technology was implemented.

Sir Godfrey Hounsfield was a farm boy who always followed his own inclinations and was never interested in going to college. He experimented with electronics as a hobby. He wrote about himself, "The period between my eleventh and eighteenth years remains the most vivid in my memory because it was the time of my first attempt at experimentation, which might never have been made had I lived in a city. In a village there are few distractions and no pressure to join in at a ball game or go to a cinema and I was free to follow a trail of any interesting idea that came my way." He worked as a radar mechanic and later studied electronic and mechanical engineering. Interested in music, he joined the research staff at EMI, the British multinational recording and publishing company, in 1951. The company also manufactured electronic devices. He made advances in computer memory design, and in 1967 moved to the central research lab of EMI and into the field of automatic pattern recognition, where he realized that much information was being lost because of inefficient data-retrieval methods.

The brilliant young man, who had an unusually powerful imagination and an everlasting wandering mind, developed the principle of three-dimensional reconstruction and thus the initial theory of computerized tomography using x-ray beams and computer technology. EMI showed no interest in Godfrey's research; they were only concerned with the manufacturing of records and music electronic components, and none of their people had any experience with radiological equipment. This extremely important device "CT scanner" would not have come to being for the medical field if it weren't for two radiologists, Dr. James Ambrose and Dr. Louis Kreel, who approached the Department of Health and Social Security to support the project. The Beatles, who recorded their songs under the EMI label, provided the most significant financial input for its advancement. Starting in 1972, the human skull was no longer a barrier for diagnosing brain conditions. Since that time, the pneumoencephalogram, a procedure that entailed replacing some cerebrospinal fluid in the brain and spinal cord with air or oxygen to improve x-ray contrast, a method in use since 1918 to diagnose brain lesions, became a thing of the past. Isn't it amazing how music lovers Thomas Edison and The Beatles contributed to ultrasound and CT, two of the most important technologies in modern medicine? However, statisticians are discouraging the excessive use of these diagnostic procedures because they necessitate excessive exposure to irradiation. It is estimated that seventy-two million scans were performed in United States in 2007, and one study estimates that as many as 0.4 percent of cancers diagnosed in this country might be from repeated scans performed earlier, and this may increase over time. Repeated studies show that radiation can cause DNA damage, and there is evidence that radiation exposure has a linear relationship with cancer. Evidence also shows that there is a significant association with the dose and that there also is a cumulative effect; however, no minimal safe dose or maximum toxic dose has been established. It has also been proven that kidney problems may happen more frequently because of the intravenous contrast material used during the procedure. Therefore, unnecessary CT scans should be avoided.

Anytime there is even a minor problem with a certain technology, scientists look for improvements and better techniques; therefore, magnetic resonance imaging (MRI) was developed as the most recent diagnostic tool, even though it does not totally replace ultrasound or CT scans. The foundation of the MRI technique began in 1946, when the phenomenon of magnetic resonance was discovered. The resonance "tendency to oscillate with greater amplitude" of electrons, atoms, molecules, or nuclei to radiation as a result of quantization in a magnetic field was only used in chemical and physical analytical procedures at first. In the early 1970s, it was shown that magnetic resonance could differentiate between normal tissue and tumors in mice. Research showed that tumors contain more water and therefore contain more hydrogen atoms and atomic nuclei, which show their presence in tissues by absorbing or emitting radio waves when exposed to a magnetic field; the availability of computers at the time made it possible for magnetic resonance to be developed into images.

The advent of superconductors that produced a strong magnetic field made it possible in 1973 to produce the first nuclear magnetic resonance image. (The conductor produces magnetism in the body, stimulates the body with radio waves to change the steady-state orientation of protons, "the positively charged particles within the atomic nuclei," and then it registers the body's electromagnetic transmissions, and these signals are used to construct images by computerized axial tomography.) The strength of the magnetic field measured by the tesla unit was proclaimed in 1956, although Nikola Tesla had discovered the rotating magnetic field back in 1882. In 1977, Paul Lauterbur from Illinois and Sir Peter Mansfield of Nottingham performed the first human MRI exam, and now the industry produces over two thousand MRI units per year, 40 percent of which are for usage in the United States. The most recent development, the functional MRI (fMRI) can read how a human's mind deals with outside stimuli and inner feelings. It maps the brain during different circumstances and will definitely help in focusing treatment on a localized affected region. The advantage of MRI is that no irradiation is involved; claustrophobic patients may have a problem with the procedure, they can be sedated or try for the more recent open MRI

The extensive improvements in medical diagnostics and many other aspects in the medical field are clearly due to the advent of IT (information technology) and ICT (information and communications technology). This reminds me of the simple communication system that was introduced to make sure the doctor was available to answer a patient's immediate needs. In the past, one would dial the phone number for the doctor's office and may or may not get an answer. The doctor exchange system was then developed to act like a centralized telephone station; the patient would call the exchange, and the operator, in turn, called the doctor. The medical professional might answer immediately, after a while, or sometimes as late as the following day. The pager system was then developed to be used inside the hospital in the form of an overhead loudspeaker, wherein everybody heard name after name of the doctors being called; this method was very disturbing to hospitalized patients. Outside the hospital, doctors carried pagers all the time to receive messages broadcast on a specific frequency over a network of radio-based stations. The problem was that some worked only in a range of twenty-five miles. The one-way pagers allowed the doctor to receive the message, but he or she needed to find a telephone to respond. (Cell phones were not available at the time.) Two-way pagers were more sophisticated, and doctors were able to send a message back. All that has changed, and with the simplification of electronic communication, doctors have the privilege to trust their patients with their e-mail address or accept text messages and answer them on the spot.

IBM produced the data management system in the 1960s and facilitated storage and retrieval of large amounts of data, and in 1981, its introduction of the personal computer (PC) gave a big boost to the application of IT with the use of computers and telecommunications equipment to store, retrieve, transmit, and manipulate data. In medicine, IT was used to automatically pro-vide patient and other information to assist in decision making, to easily connect doctors with their clients, and to increase efficiency. Senator Edward Kennedy was, for a long time, deeply involved in trying to make improvements in the health-care system in the United States. He was interested in implementing cost sav-ings, and he realized that the medical profession relied on intense information communication; this was when the potential of IT was considered by insurance companies for collecting patient information and by medical record departments to store infor-mation electronically. Medical information could be condensed into a single database and retrieved with a click of a mouse. Of course, patient privacy advocates got involved; they felt that col-lecting patient data was unethical in regard to the doctor-patient relationship and that the practice exposed confidential patient information to insurance companies. There was also worry about errors in data entry that might be difficult to correct, so the idea was abandoned at the time. Senator Kennedy could not get a bill passed, and information technology could not be used for patient data collection. However, it was used tremendously in pharma-ceuticals; hospital pharmacies and general ones implemented IT; it kept track of drug usage, minimized patient wait times for medication, prevented prescription duplication, and reduced the danger of drug interaction.

When we introduced IT in our hospital laboratory in the early 1980s, it was a big ordeal. We had to provide training sessions for the doctors, and many of them were not computer savvy yet and resented the change. They preferred to look at paper records and printed results rather than using a computer, typing in their ID and user number or password, and searching for the reports. After training, doctors were thankful and appreciative when they were able to get their patients' laboratory results that were available electronically rather than waiting for the reports to be typed and sent to them. In those days, hospitals could only afford to provide one computer in the nursing station of each ward, and doctors had to wait for their turn to use it; that was the only drawback and waste of time. Things changed over the years, though; amazingly, when one walks along hospital corridors now, one can often observe nurses sitting outside each patient's room at a small desk with a computer, entering patient's data and information. It is also not uncommon to visit a doctor's office, and he or she comes into the examination room to see you, carrying a laptop or tablet that contains all the patient information he or she needs, and it saves a lot of time traditionally needed for questions. I recently heard on the business financial news that the year 2014 saw an explosion of investment in IT related to the health industry.

Automation is another scientific development that brought extensive improvements to the medical practice. When I was working on my thesis for my doctoral degree, in the early 1960s, part of the research process required me to investigate structural and functional changes in the liver and run tests (liver profiles) on my patients before and after the new modes of treatment I administered and to tabulate and compare the results. It took me two days just to add reagents to the patients' blood to perform each test separately for every patient, to get the results of the transaminases. I needed to collect blood in several test tubes for each patient separately, in certain amounts, and I added multiple reagents with pipettes one by one, each for a certain period of time waiting for the chemical reaction to happen. If any of the amounts was not exact, I got inaccurate results and had to repeat the whole procedure. About ten years later, in the mid-1970s, I was director of a hospital laboratory, and much had changed. We worked with a Coulter counter and a biochemical analyzer that were fully automated. A few drops of blood were delivered from measuring cups at one end of the machine, and the results appeared for all the patients tested together at the other end in less than half an hour. Physicians were amazed at the speed with which they could get printed reports.

Another ten years later, because of ongoing research and development in the field of clinical laboratories, things changed again. The notable development in this case was the number of new tests that could be performed and how their results were interpreted. For example, cholesterol of three hundred milligrams per deciliter in the blood was considered to be normal; patients were advised to adopt exercise and a healthy diet to lower it by 10 to 20 percent if found to be higher till it was proven statistically that some people with this level of cholesterol developed heart attacks, so the desired normal level of cholesterol was reduced from three hundred to two hundred milligrams per deciliter. This level is difficult to sustain without the use of statin medications such as Lipitor, Zocor, or Crestor, with or without the consideration of other risk factors such as stress, diabetes, and high blood pressure. Similar developments took place with blood glucose testing, the evaluation for diabetes. The fasting normal level of glucose in the blood has been lowered also from one hundred to seventy milligrams per deciliter. In other words, what used to be considered normal is now labeled prediabetic, and those people are advised to watch their carbohydrate intake in their diet and may be given some oral medication. A new test was added (HA1C) to measure the mean blood glucose level during the previous three months, so patients cannot trick doctors by watching their diet for a couple of days before having their fasting level tested.

You can't feel or see osteoporosis, and it therefore used to be called the silent disease. However, the advent of the densitometer makes detecting this disease much easier. One can now see it, and it is treated even though you cannot feel it to prevent its complication of fractures. In fact, people are advised to start treatment at an earlier stage, when a bone minimal density test diagnoses them with osteopenia rather than full blown osteoporosis. Before this test was available, the patient's blood calcium level was measured during the yearly checkup; if found to be low, the patient was recommended supplements to keep healthy bones. Recently, a test for vitamin D gained popularity as a routine measurement, even though its level in the blood is not yet standardized. Everybody I know is taking calcium and vitamin D, but to attain my normal level of the latter, I just roll up my sleeves, elevate my skirt a little, and sit in the sun.

The people who are interested in the recent history of medical technology increasingly attend the International Trade Fair and Congress for Medical Technology and the exhibits of the World Forum for Medicine in Dusseldorf, Germany. Wolfgang Albath, a pioneer in laboratory medicine, was one of the founding organizers of the show MEDICA, which started in Karlsruhe, Germany, in 1969. The Technicon AutoAnalyzer, which we used in our laboratory, was first demonstrated at this trade show. The immunofluorescent technique, whereby a fluorescence microscope is used to visualize a specific antibody antigen response assisted by the addition of a fluorescent dye and thus identify the antigen, was also introduced there. Albath, proud of his involvement in laboratory technology, said, "Recent history can be described in three words,

Mechanization, Automation and Digitalization." The way he described advancements in surgical techniques like keyhole surgery, meaning laparoscopy, was interesting, and he referred to the use of laser by saying, "It lit up the medical sky." Ira Brodsky's work also provides tremendous information about recent advances. He has thirty years of experience bringing new technology to life. He was president of Datacomm Research for nineteen years. His book The History of Wireless explains how creative minds, inventors, and entrepreneurs produced technology for the masses and energized the market for wireless. Another of his books, *The History and Future of Medical Technology* tells the story behind advanced medical technologies: how they developed, how they work, and how they are likely to evolve in the coming years; the future is unbelievably glamorous. The Technicon Corporation has another dream for the near future: They are in the process of developing InSightec for the future operating room so that surgeries could be performed noninvasively—without cutting at all. The InSightec device will allow the use of ultrasound through an electronically controlled transducer and, with the application of a combination of physics, mathematics, ultrasound, and electronics, reach the diseased part inside the body and eradicate it.

A PEEK INTO THE FUTURE

I have a granddaughter who is interested in medicine, but she would prefer to be a veterinarian than a medical doctor. When she was ten years old, she told me this was because "animals are easier to work with; they do not ask questions and are obedient pets." She has a dog and a cat and enjoys horseback riding. She is also very interested in technology and spends much of her time playing games on her iPhone and working with her iPad. She said, "I cannot wait to see how technology will develop during the coming ten years and how this progress will affect the world." I share her thoughts, especially relative to health care and how new developments in technology are going to affect the field. While surfing the Internet together, my granddaughter and I ran across a site that attracted our attention. It said, "St. Joseph Health: Robotic and Minimally Invasive Treatment." These types of treatments are a big part of the future of medicine, including the next generation of surgery and how the little girl's dad will conduct his work. Like we did in the past, a surgeon introduces him- or herself to the patient in the same way we used to do and then examines the patient thoroughly, explains the recommended procedure, and gets the required consent. The doctor accompanies the patient to the operating room and makes sure he or she is lying comfortably on the operating table; then, however, the surgeon turns away from the patient and goes to work on a console with a computer screen. A robot actually performs the procedure, while the surgeon directs it by telemanipulation, the procedure is also defined as remote surgery, where the surgeon is the master and the robot is the slave.

The Lindbergh Operation, well known among physicians, was the first successful remote surgery, performed in 2001. By that time, minimally invasive surgery was well-established. Camera guidance and the introduction of computer-assisted procedures, wherein artificial intelligence enhanced the safety of the surgeon's movements, were utilized; the concept of a distance between the surgeon and the patient was also well understood. The operation was not named after the surgeon who performed the surgery as usual, but after the American aviator Charles Lindbergh, who was the first person to make a nonstop long-distance solo flight across the Atlantic Ocean from Paris to NewYork. A team of French surgeons in New York performed the operation on a patient in Strasbourg, France, by telesurgery over a distance of several thousand miles across the same ocean. The transatlantic computer-assisted robotic minimally invasive laparoscopic cholecystectomy that was performed was successful.

For a long time, NASA funded robotic research and techniques to service the satellites from the ground rather than sending somebody into space. It is said that the word "robot" was first introduced in the year 1921 by the Czech writer Karel Capek, in his play *R.U.R. (Rossum's Universal Robots)* about compulsory labor, but the idea had been entertained and applied many years before. Aristotle, the great philosopher wrote in 322 BCE, "If every tool when ordered or even of its own accord, could do the work that befits it, then there would be no need either of apprentices for the master workers or slaves." Many years later, the idea was introduced for entertainment. Leonardo da Vinci designed the armored knight to amuse royalty around the 1490s. Jacques de Vaucanson presented life-size automatons, The Flute Player and The Tambourine, in the late 1730s, during a period of craze for animation; his most important development was a duck he called "moving anatomy"; it could flap its wings and quack. In 1770, the Swiss watchmaker Pierre Jaquet-Droz invented clocks that interacted with moving dolls. The aforementioned examples were not useful robots, but they represented the fantasy of initiating different movements in nonliving objects. Fritz Lang, the German filmmaker, produced several silent movies. The most famous one was titled *Metropolis*, meant to represent futuristic science fiction, wherein a female robot played a role. Issac Asimov, the professor of biochemistry in Boston, was also interested in mysteries, fantasy, and science fiction. In 1940, he published several storybooks, including a series about robots.

Robots later moved from fiction to reality; the first documented use of a robot assisting in a surgical procedure was in 1985, when the PUMA 560 was used to accurately place a needle to obtain a brain biopsy with CT guidance. In 1988, doctors used the PROBOT to perform successful prostatic surgery. Year after year, improvements were made, and different settings were used. In 1992, the ROBODOC was introduced and used for hip replacement. Robotic endoscopic procedures were not approved by the FDA until 1990. The da Vinci Surgical System for laparoscopic surgery was approved in the year 2000; a surgeon controlled the device from a console, and the system included a patient-side cart with four interactive arms, also controlled from the console, and an endoscopic camera. It is estimated that as of January 2013, more than two thousand units have been sold all over the world.

General surgeons are discussing the dilemma regarding the future of robotics. Some do not consider robotic surgery to be the only or best minimally invasive approach for certain surgeries; others are of the opinion that there is no way back from robotics.

Benefits and challenges are still being discussed, and yet (Intuit Surgical Inc) the company that markets the da Vinci system claims that requests for their product are steadily increasing. In addition, reports addressing the outcome of surgical procedures demonstrate that approaches using robotics is as good as, and even better than laparoscopic approaches without its use. The surgeon is able to see three-dimensional images, and surgeon hand tremor is eliminated, giving him or her more ease and precision during the procedure. The dilemma arises in the cost, the need for new policies and standards for using robotics, and the complexity it brings to the environment of the operating room. However, hospitals are marketing robotics as evidence that they are the state-of-the-art facilities. As of December 2012, financial analysts were recommending that investors buy and hold stock in Intuitive Surgical, leading one to conclude that there will be a great need for robots. In fact, the latest use of robots in hospitals is as a combatant of bacteria. The TRU-D device is a five-foot-five robot that emits ultraviolet rays lethal to resistant hospital-based infectious organisms; it is used to disinfect patient rooms and surgery suites. There are already more than one hundred in use in hospitals and medical facilities.

Implants, hair, teeth, lens, were not a big deal. Joint replacements were a form of implants that took years for the medical field to perfect. Early problems have practically been eliminated for the future. In Germany, T. Gluck experimented in 1891 with implanting an ivory femoral head for hip replacement, but it failed. In 1940, Dr. Austin Moore performed the first metallic hip-joint replacement using Vitallium, a cobalt-chrome alloy; this method also proved to have problems, even though it was improved upon in 1952. Orthopedic surgeons went back to using ivory, but there were always problems with joint-surface lubrication, instability, and infection. Since 1970, stainless steel, polyethylene, bone cement, and synovial fluid lubrication solved the old problems and perfected hip replacement. Dr. Theophilus Gluck also experimented with knee-joint replacement; to reduce friction, he tried to cushion the joint surfaces with muscle, fat, nylon, and other materials, but none of them worked. Finally, the idea of a rotating joint replaced the old weight-bearing fixed joint, and since the late 1990s, a minimally invasive technique is being used; it allows faster recovery, less pain, and fewer complications.

Regenerative medicine, wherein scientists and bioengineers are in the process of creating organs to be regrown from patient's stem cells, to be available for later transplants, is an emerging field that has made tremendous advancements since I was in school and practicing medicine. Stem cells are undifferentiated cells that can divide and differentiate into specialized cell types; they are able to self-renew indefinitely in culture media to produce more stem cells. They are either embryonic stem cells, obtained from early-stage embryos, or adult stem cells, obtained from skin, bone, marrow, blood, fat cells, or an umbilical cord. Centers dealing with regenerative medicine and stem-cell research conduct a revolutionary exploration of human disease in addition to organ transplants. Through these efforts, in addition to the personalized stem-cell-based therapies, the future of cancer care became very promising.

The theory of transplants has been studied for quite some time and repeatedly attempted. Rhinoplasty (plastic surgery on the nose) was one of the first attempts of allografted skin transplants, but it was not successful; the patient's body rejected the transplanted skin, so it fell off. The first successful allograft (a transplant from a genetically nonidentical donor to a recipient without producing an immune response or rejection), was a corneal transplant of an eye, performed in 1837. The cornea is avascular, meaning it has no blood supply, and this might have been the reason for its success. In 1882, thyroid glandular tissue could be implanted into patients who needed it because their own gland was dysfunctional and could not produce enough of the hormone. In the twentieth century, arteries and veins could be taken from donors and sutured to those in a patient.

Blood transfusion was one of the first methods of transferring tissue from a normally healthy person to a needy patient. It took years of experimenting after 1874 until scientists realized that sodium citrate, an anticoagulant, needed to be added to prevent the transfused blood from clotting. The blood needed to be refrigerated and kept at a certain temperature all the time, and it needed to be obtained from a specific donor; otherwise, it would sometimes cause serious side effects, even death. Most of the time, it caused chills, fever, and dark urine because the recipient's body was breaking down the blood cells. This caused doctors to realize that the blood had to be compatible to prevent this breaking-down process—that is, it had to be from a person of the same "ABO group and RH factor." Blood transfusion problems were easily solved, but with transfusions of bone marrow and other tissues, it was not that simple; factors other than the ABO/RH compatibility had to be considered. Newton's third law of motion says, "For every action there is a reaction equal to it and opposite in direction." Our bodies work in a similar manner, so for every foreign body (antigen) introduced into the body, there develops a specific antibody that reacts to it, leading to what is called, "graft versus host disease." Our immune mechanism responds and rejects the substance that has been introduced. There has to be histocompatibility between a donor and the recipient host to prevent rejection during any tissue or organ transplant. In the year 1958, an antigen was detected to be present on human white blood cells, the HLA, or human leukocyte antigen; it was the basis for histocompatibility, and since that time, tremendous research and development has been done in the field of organ transplant by identifying the antigen-antibody immune complex.

The discovery of the immunosuppressant drug cyclosporine, which suppresses such rejection, was another breakthrough event. This substance was obtained from a fungus in 1969, and the practice of transplantation moved from experimentation to human surgical procedures. Other immunosuppressants are presently in use. Dr. Denton Cooley in Houston, Texas, pioneered heart transplants in humans in the United States in 1968. (At the time when my husband worked with him as a fellow in 1964, Dr. Cooley had not yet started this amazing work.) His claim to fame at that time was the tremendous improvements he made to the heart-lung machine used for open-heart surgery. During 1968, Dr. Cooley performed seventeen of these cardiac procedures, including the first transplant of both heart and lungs, but the median life span after surgery was only six months. During Dr. Cooley's career as a cardiac surgeon, he and his associates reportedly performed more than 118,800 surgeries, more than any other cardiac team in the world. However, in 1967, Christian Barnard had performed the very first heart transplant, in Cape Town, South Africa, after he had experimented with fifty transplants on dogs. The surgery is said to have lasted for nine, hours, and he used a team of thirty people; his patient only lived for eighteen days afterward. Techniques and results improved in 1984, and there was a 65 percent five-year survival rate for transplant patients. Organ transplantation soon became a routine surgical procedure with long-term survival rates for the kidneys, heart, liver, lungs, and pancreas as well as for limbs and partial-face procedures. It is clear that autografts ("self that is from a person to himself") and isografts ("from a genetically identical donor") are less risky and not as prone to rejection as other circumstances.

It was in fact Dr. Michael DeBakey (Figure 21) who made Houston, Texas, a major center for heart surgery and research and turned Baylor University into one of the nation's great medical centers, and my husband worked with him. He had a short stature, a dark complexion, an intelligent look, piercing eyes, and a striking presence and influence. Residents and fellows in his department competed to work with him and to assist him so they could learn his new techniques. They even rushed to get into the operating room before him, so they had to be scrubbed by five in the morning. Dr. DeBakey was a Lebanese immigrant, and he credited much of his surgical skill to his mother, Raheeja, who taught him to sew, crochet, and knit. He produced many innovations and worked very hard, starting his day early. In 2006, when he underwent surgery to repair a torn aorta, a surgical procedure he had devised fifty years earlier preserved his own life. He traveled a lot and was recognized all over the world for his achievements. He recently passed away at the age of ninety-nine, from natural causes, at the same hospital where he had saved the lives of thousands of patients.

In my own field of medicine, pathology, the future will differ a great deal from the past. This science was deemed in the late 1920s to be a medical specialty with two major departments: anatomic pathology, examining organs, tissues, and cells, and clinical pathology, which is laboratory work. It had been a subject of interest to doctors since the nineteenth century, but it was not fully understood or developed. It was referred to as "morbid anatomy" to differentiate between normal (healthy) and diseased tissue as seen by the naked eye or under the light microscope. However, Rudolf Virchow (1821–1902) the German anthropologist, biologist, politician, prehistorian, and pathologist, known as the father of pathology, theorized and proved that disease affects organs and tissues on a cellular level. After so many years, the future of pathology depends on this theory of cellular and specifically intra-cellular changes.

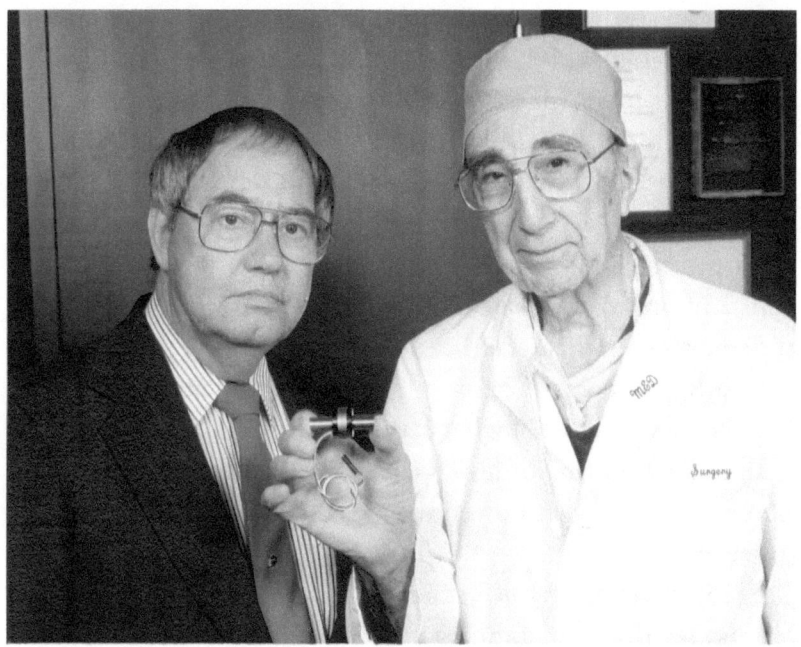

FIGURE 21

Molecular pathology is an emerging discipline, adopted mainly by oncologists to help cancer patients and in cytogenetic testing. This new branch of science has been in the forefront of laboratory medicine since its inception in 1989. It arrived shortly after the PCR (polymerase chain reaction) became standardized. PCR is a biochemical technology in molecular biology through which one can amplify one or more copies of a piece of DNA and copy it across several orders of magnitude a billion times. By amplification, the minute details of cells can be visualized, DNA can be decoded, and sequencing can be easily performed. It is a relatively simple and inexpensive tool used in diagnosing hereditary diseases or dealing with genetic problems. Kary Mullis, a Nobel Prize–winning American biochemist developed this technique in 1983. Molecular pathology focuses on studying and diagnosing disease through examination of the molecules within organs, tissues, and body fluids. It combines molecular and genetic approaches to diagnose and classify tumors, and it validates the prediction of biomarkers in a patient's tissues that indicate progression of disease and regression due to treatment response. The discipline also identifies the susceptibility of individuals of different genetic constitutions to develop cancer and the environmental and lifestyle factors implicated in carcinogenesis. This emerging field is creating a new paradigm in disease treatment; methods are based on knowledge of what causes a particular disease, paired with understanding of how we can leverage the individual patient's cells to control or eliminate the disease and regenerate diseased organs.

Molecular testing is fast becoming standard in clinical laboratory testing, and pathologists who trained to use it are doing a great favor to their clinician colleagues and their patients. For example, when statistical studies of patients were analyzed, it was found that treatment decisions for the patients for whom the molecular testing was performed had to be changed according to the analyses results 45 percent of the time; and recommendation for chemotherapy fell from 52 percent pretest to 30 percent afterward. Sometime during the nineteenth century, Mendel predicted the existence of genes theoretically (he did not name his findings genes), but they were later proven to be true. We studied the Mendel principle of heredity in biology class at my high school. However, all we understood at the time was that such inherited characteristics as blue eyes, black hair, stature, and weight are transmitted in a family tree among the members in a predictable way for several generations, depending on whether the characteristic is a dominant or recessive trait. Mendel practiced genetic engineering; today, this practice is a health issue of concern. It is under debate and has been put on several voting ballots. The public requested a ruling by the FDA to label all foods that have been genetically engineered, not realizing that most of them are. Mendel grew peas in his garden, and he noticed the effect of crossing different strains of the plant and how the offspring acquired characteristics from both original plants. The Mendel principle was not further scientifically researched till the discovery of deoxyribonucleic acid, or DNA (figure 22) ; this discovery made the field of genetics explode. A gene is a length of DNA strands that contains the instructions to make chemicals in the body and codes for a protein. Proteins are complex forms of amino acids coded as A for Adenine, T for thymine, C for cytosine, G for guanine, and U for uracil. These combine in different sequences to form complete sets of instructions to make each individual cell in the body; the set of instructions is called the genome.

When my son graduated from college, he had majored in biochemistry and taken a master's degree in physiology, two great science fields that made contributions to medicine. I tried to persuade him to find a job in one of these two progressive fields, but he preferred to pursue his career in medicine as a surgeon. If he had listened, he might be working on a research project of the future of medicine rather than working with robotics and computers. Techniques of biochemistry, molecular biology, and genetics are applied in proteomics, a futuristic branch of biotechnology. It is concerned with analyzing the structure, functions, and interactions of the proteins produced by the genes of a particular cell,

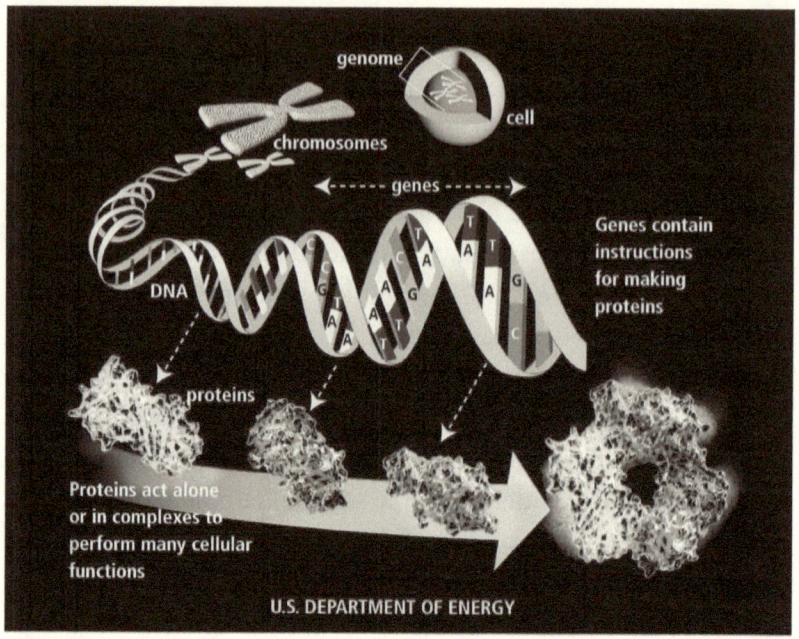

FIGURE 22

tissue, or organism and organizing the information into a database for future use. The term "proteomics" was coined in 1997, the same year I retired from working as a pathologist. Therefore, I never studied it or ran any of its tests; all my knowledge about it is from keeping up with medical journals and a continuous medical education and I find it fascinating. This advanced method of testing was named proteomics (the study of proteins, the building blocks to life) to form an analogy with genomics (the study of genes). However, there is a big difference: An organism's genes are more or less constant, whereas a proteome differs from cell to cell and from time to time; there are also transitional modifications. Our DNA is static, but our proteins are dynamic. Proteins are the main components of the physiological metabolic pathways of cells—that is, the chemical reactions within each cell that often need minerals and vitamins as a cofactor to keep "homeostasis" and "equilibrium and stability." In other words, they need to stay healthy and maintain a balance between catabolism, "breaking down," and anabolism, "synthesis and building up" pathways, which are the step-by-step modification of an initial molecule to be used immediately, to initiate another metabolic pathway, or to be stored by the cell for further use. Proteins are part of the structure of enzymes, catalysts, immune-response mechanisms, cell adhesiveness, and the structure of all muscles; proteins, particularly the essential amino acids that our body cannot process, are necessary for growth. Therefore, it is of utmost importance to include them in our food, because we are what we eat. It is estimated that there are twenty thousand to twenty-five thousand proteins in the body, and this number may increase drastically in the near future. Due to the process of slicing and transformational modification, their number may soon reach one million, which could further complicate these studies. Deciphering the genetic basis of disease has been a great challenge for many years, yet tests using DNA sequencing is now a great tool used to improve diagnosis and treatment of genetic disorders. The conventional Sanger sequencer was the first generation of technology applied; it was developed by Frederick Sanger in 1977 and has since been used for approximately twenty-five years. It produced 0.06 megabytes of data at a cost of 1,500 dollars per megabyte. The next-generation sequencer can now produce six hundred thousand megabytes of data at a cost of four cents per megabyte, and it only takes fifteen minutes to sequence a human genome; what was once unthinkable in the diagnosis, prognosis, and treatment of diseases is now achievable. Soon, personalized medicine based on next-generation sequencing is on its way to making a dream come true; individual metrics will become each person's advocate for his or her well-being.

With all these advances, I would like to return to Newton's third law: "For every action there is a reaction." World events act similarly but not to the same extent or in the exact same manner as in the realm of physics. So, for many discoveries, there is a reaction and the pros and cons. For example, the discovery of vaccines was one of the cornerstones in public health improvement. Every child and adult was immunized to improve child mortality and reduce epidemics, particularly in third-world and developing countries. However, this did not go hand in hand with improved education and a higher standard of living; the result was overcrowding and an increased population dealing with poverty and famine. The discovery of antibiotics proved a great success and fought a war against bacteria, tremendously reducing the death rate from infection, but because people overused and abused this method, the bugs fought back. They mutated and developed resistance, some to the extent that they do not respond to antibiotics anymore, as in the case of the well-known bacteria MRSA (Methicillin-resistant Staphylococcus aureus). There is no way to get rid of this bacteria strain with our present knowledge, because a mutation is a permanent change in the DNA sequence of a gene, and it forms a totally different kind that would not respond to the antibiotic similarly to the original bacteria. The amino acid sequence of a protein is altered, a change that can lead to virulent organisms. The same thing happens with viruses that sometimes lead to severe flu epidemics. The mutation of a particular gene is known to lead to a predisposition for cancer, but mutation also occurs in the cancer cells themselves when treated with chemotherapy; therefore we see more leukemia develop in patients treated for breast cancer. In addition, mutation of a particular gene will predispose a person to some kind of disease other than cancer.

Most drugs have tradeoffs and shift the balance of homeostasis one way or another, leading to undesired side effects. Side effects of drugs are a well-known occurrence; the system in the body targeted with the medicine will respond favorably, and the specific disease is alleviated, while other systems or organs may react neg-atively to the same medicine. It is frequently not very clear how in-dividual bodies will respond or react to a certain drug; it depends on the person's immune response. Numerous studies are still in progress to identify paradoxes of the overuse of vitamins and the balance between using antioxidants and their paradoxical effect on the normal oxidation process in the body, the basis for energy production. Medications can cause other types of negative unex-pected results. For example, reactions to vaccinations have caused children to die, and patients allergic to penicillin were killed by an injection of the antibiotic. After Viagra was introduced to the public as a wonder drug, it caused heart attacks in some patients. The anti-inflammatory drugs Vioxx and Celebrex acted like magic to alleviate pain, but both of them caused heart attacks or strokes, and Vioxx had to be withdrawn from the market. Tragedy struck when thalidomide was prescribed as a tranquilizer for pregnant women in 1964; it had a good effect, but no one knew at the time that it caused severe birth defects in their offspring.

Computer technology enhanced the medical practice as well, yet incidental findings of no significance are a thing of the past. With the help of CT and MRI these so-called incidental find-ings are investigated and properly diagnosed, many times at a high cost, not to mention causing inconvenience and worry for the patient, and ultimately failing to produce helpful results. All additional diagnostic investigations may turn out to be negative and sometimes are risky for the patient leading to undesired con-cequences. Ultrasound and CT scans are great diagnostic tools, yet as aforementioned, they may cause excessive exposure to irra-diation and might be carcinogenic to some individuals; dyes used for contrast may cause kidney failure.

When you have trouble with your car, you take it to a me-chanic who will fix it or replace a part; the car is manmade. When something goes wrong at your home, you ask a builder for help, and he or she will easily take care of it. When your faucet leaks, your neighborhood plumber will help you mend it. When you lose money, you get a financial advisor's assistance. But when your body or one of your organs loses one of its normal functions, you do not know where to start. Doctors and researchers still have not entirely figured out how our creator made us out of many very minute (or invisible) intricate, interconnected, and interactive parts that need nanosensors to detect and fix. In spite of all the medical innovations, doctors and researchers are still looking at the human body like a book that has been opened, but the pages have not been fully read yet; in many ways, they are still shooting in the dark.

In spite of the negative examples mentioned in this chapter, I foresee an attractive future. The CDC and WHO statistics tell me that the fertility rate, currently a report on the number of live births per ten thousand women between the ages of fifteen and forty-four, is improving; the high end of the age range will definitely be raised in the future. The premature mortality rate that reflects the number of deaths among people younger than age seventy-five per one hundred thousand residents is also improving and expected to improve more in the future. Even though, in the view of these organizations, the aforementioned types of deaths affecting mortality rates depend 30 percent on genetics and 70 percent on lifestyle—the type of food one eats, exercise one gets, smoking habits, and more—improvement in health services has recently made a great impact. I can see a future where there will be less lobbying by the drug businesses and insurance companies and more lobbying for new technology to facilitate better health screening, increased preventive methods, and more spending on personal and individualized medical care, rather than drugs and hospitals.

And now I can tell my curious granddaughter that I imagine a future where babies can easily be made in test tubes and then implanted into the mother's womb, whatever age the woman is; a woman will be able to choose whether she becomes pregnant with a boy or a girl. I can see a world where everybody is vaccinated, and every patient can receive a proper antibiotic, so there will be no reason to die from an infection. In the future, tumors can be detected early enough for eradication before they even start growing, and with the aid of proteomics, doctors can know in advance who is prone to be affected with cancer and prevent the cancer from happening at all. I imagine a world where lenses and hearing aids can restore senses, a world where rusty joints can be replaced and where failed internal organs like the heart, lung, kidney, or liver can be transplanted with no side effects or rejection. I foresee a time where there will be a global melting pot of everybody's health data, whether each person is healthy or sick; this information will include proteomics and genomics so that doctors do not have to spend time taking a history or doing a physical. They will simply go to a website, type in their ID and password, and retrieve patient information to start individualized preventive measures and personalized treatments accordingly. There will also come a day when a patient is sent for surgery to a nearby hospital, and that person's surgeon goes to a central robotics computer lab to perform the procedure with minimal invasion as well as reduced pain and discomfort to the patient, no matter what the geographical distance between them is. Patients can travel, knowing that their local doctor can still communicate in case of emergency, and a telesurgery can be performed. Finally, in this future, an aged person can appear ten, twenty, or even thirty years younger with the help of plastic surgery, Botox and implants. There will be no children left to die, no organs left to fail, and no growing people left to age. Isn't that eternity—but at what cost will we attain it?

AT WHAT COST

The lowest cost of health care to the patient was during the time when the patient went to see a family doctor and relied totally on that professional's judgment and advice and then paid the physician a fee for taking good care of him. A version of this system was discussed briefly in a previous chapter. I can attest to the fact that when the patient needed to be referred to one or more specialists, the fees would double or triple; when lab tests were required, the charges would increase further, but not much, because there weren't that many tests to be performed or diagnostic tools available to be used. There were not many choices of medicines for treatment either, but the cost of treatment rose tremendously when the patient was finally hospitalized or needed surgery, and that did not occur very often.

When I was a little girl, I was happy to see my dad come home, smiling, and say, "I did well for my patients and for myself today." He counted the bills in his wallet and then gave me some cash to buy something for myself. He kept a log in his office of his receivables and expenses. The fees for his services were not fixed; instead, they depended on how his patients felt when their health improved and how much they valued his efforts. When my peers and I went into private practice several years later, physicians still made their living through a fee for services. There were no set fees, but patients paid their doctors according to some agreed-upon facts determined by the extent of their sickness, how involved the doctor would be, and the doctor's reputation and position in the community. A university professor was known to charge the highest fees; a surgeon charged more than a general practitioner; and a hospital admission raised the cost. Government hospitals were always available for the poor, where all services were free.

The fee-for-service model is not a modern way of dealing; it was mentioned in The Code of Hammurabi during the Babylonian era, circa 1772 BCE. It was meant to be a code of justice and is considered the oldest well-preserved code of law, produced and enacted by the sixth Babylonian king (Iraqi, in terms of present-day geography); archeologists excavated it in 1901. It is written on a human-sized stone and clay tablets, and it involves all aspects of life. It has apparent similarity to the laws of Moses, later revised in the Hebrew Bible and named The Ten Commandments. The commandment regarding an eye for an eye is a paraphrase of one of the laws from the Code of Hammurabi considered to be related to any type of malpractice.

The relevant segment of the Hammurabi code says the following:

> *If a surgeon has operated with the bronze lancet on a Patrician for a serious injury and has cured him, or has removed with his bronze lancet a cataract for a patrician and has cured his eye, he shall take ten shekels of silver. If it be a plebeian he shall take five shekels of silver, if it be a man's slave he the owner of the slave shall give the five silver shekels. If a surgeon has operated with his bronze lancet on a patrician for a serious injury and has caused his death or has removed a cataract for a patrician with a bronze lancet and has made him lose his eye, his hands shall be cut off.*

The code also mentions how to pay for a slave's death and that if a slave loses an eye, the owner should be paid for half the slave's value. The code of law regarded the whole population of men as falling into three classes: the *amelu*, the *muskinu*, and the *ardu*. The amelu (patrician) was the family man whose birth, marriage, and death were marked with ancestral estates and full civil rights. This type of man had aristocratic privileges and responsibilities, and he had the right to retaliation for corporal injury as well as liability to heavier punishment, higher fees, and fines to pay. The andu was a slave, and the muskanu was a beggar, poor or landless.

In the early 1960s, when my husband and I left Egypt for the first-time on a one-year fellowship to Germany, we were not paid much. Our grants covered regular daily expenses, and money was scarce. I needed to be admitted to the hospital for a week, and I didn't know how I would pay for it. On discharge, I inquired about the bill, and the staff member told me that it was settled. My stipend covered me fully for physician fees, hospital charges, and all medications, with no deductable, co-payment or a dime out of pocket. It was a pleasant surprise and a relief, and at the time, I did not even question how it was possible to be given such good care for free, but now I understand how the German health system is set up. I read an article titled "National Health-Care Medicine in Germany, 1918–1945," and I started to admire their system. In the late 1960s, we settled for good in the United States, and everybody was again talking about a fee-for-service system for health care as being the best in the world. Doctor's fees were affordable, and hospital charges depended on factors as its location, members of staff and whether you stayed in a room with a double bed or a single bed or in a VIP room; labs, x-rays, and other investigative measures were also included in the hospital charges. Forty years have elapsed since then; things kept changing drastically, and the cost of health care went through the roof.

I read an interesting article published by Georgetown University, titled "The Cost of Health Care: 1958 vs. 2012." In that article, Mark Perry economist and scholar at the American Enterprise Institute, attempted to analyze and compare the cost of health care to the cost of purchasing goods and retail items, using the term "time cost." He calculated the hours of work required to purchase things and concluded that the consumer of that year, working at an average wage of $19 per hour would only have to work 26.6 hours to earn enough income ($511) to purchase a high-end toaster, TV, or iPod. The equivalent products would have required 4.64 weeks of work in the year 1958. The author therefore concluded that the time cost of these items declined 86 percent in less than five decades. He tried to apply the same analyses to health care, and his research lead him to the fact that in 1958, per capita health-care expenditure was $134, and a worker earning the average wage at the time ($1.98 per hour) would have had to work 15 days to cover this expense. By 2012, per capita health spending climbed to $8,953, and at the average wage, one had to work 58 days to cover that. These numbers revealed that by 2012, while the time cost for other goods plummeted to less than one quarter their level in 1958, the time cost for health care more than quadrupled. Perry writes that health care improved tremendously during these years, but so did the quality and performance of other goods like dishwashers and televisions, although not much technology is involved in these items. He blames this discrepancy in change over the decades on the relation between the consumer and the payer. The consumer buys goods and pays out of pocket, but for health care, a third party pays.

An updated article by Sarah Cliff about the same theory of time cost states a different view. She notes that it is much less expensive to buy a washer and dryer presently compared to the cost in 1958 because technology has not changed much. Even for those items in which technology has improved, such as an iPod compared to a four-speed record player, there is a decline in time cost. In health care, many factors play a role other than a third-party payer, including an aging population, administrative costs, advanced technology, defensive medicine, the cost of drugs, and supplier-induced demand.

An article in the *Washington Post* from March 2012, by Ezra Klein titled "Why an MRI costs $1,080 in America and $280 in France," debates several reasons for the marked difference; in fact, in the United States, some institutions charge $3,500 for a complicated MRI. It mentions that in 2009, Americans spent $7,960 per person on health, while in Canada, it was only $4,808; in Germany, $4,218 and in France, $3,978. The article contemplates several possibilities, including seeing the doctors more often, using more services, and patients' families being more demanding, but the final conclusion was that prices of goods and services are higher. There is no control; it is a free market. The MRI scanner alone used to cost over one million dollars, but it recently went down to fifty thousand dollars. And construction of MRI suites could cost up to five hundred thousand dollars. A robot used in surgery costs $2.6 million and adds $4,800 to the cost of each surgical procedure. Who pays for these costs other than the consumer?

Goods and services related to health care are plentiful. Machinery for ultrasound, x-rays, CT scanners, and MRIs improved tremendously with new technology: analyzers, now fully automated; electronics, including hardware and software; instruments; and medications. Hospitals and institutions add buildings and departments to accommodate new developments; to promote these new developments, salespeople, marketing people, and agents are needed. Most importantly, patients must have medical insurance; it goes up with age. Similarly, doctors are covered by malpractice insurance, which increases every time there is a claim.

I met a doctor practicing robotic surgery. He had just returned from a training course in a new technique developed for performing minimally invasive laparoscopic robotic surgery; the company that manufactured new instrumentation for this procedure invited him. In other words, the company is presenting its new goods, and the doctors are being trained to use them in providing their services. Recently, in a three-page article in a newspaper, a writer debates the ethics of how academics influence the use of new and expensive technological procedures like robotic surgery. She raises questions about university-based doctors' advocacy for promoting new devices, meanwhile boosting their own prestige and professional finances. It is well-known that pharmaceutical and medical-device companies recruit academics to test, investigate, give lectures on, provide training, and then recommend the use of a product. "A recommendation from a professor means much more than a pitch from a sales person." Who is better qualified to decide the benefits of using the product? This matter would only be questionable if professors received a high honorarium or compensation for travel expenses to give these lectures, even though this is normal and ethically acceptable in the field of medical devices and pharmaceuticals. It may be frowned upon when the university medical school gets a big grant for using and training their doctors on the new product, while other hospitals do not. When my fellow residents and I were approached by pharmaceutical companies to test drugs in the pipeline on government hospital patients with the approval of our professors, no grants were involved, and the products we tested were not nearly as expensive as the ones being promoted presently.

The debate now is about high-cost technology and extremely expensive machinery, prompted by the cost involved in the system. It is said that by the end of the year 2006, revenues for the manufacturer of the da Vinci robot, Intuitive, rose by more than 60 percent a year, and the company was sitting on $240 million in cash. Manufacturers of printers mainly profit from selling the ink, not the printer. Likewise, Intuitive profits in millions not only from the price of the robot, which amounts to about 2.3 million dollars, but also from selling parts that cost up to $2,200 and an annual service contract for up to $180,000. There are definite pros for using robotic surgeries to better service the patients; it is supposed to save time and reduce pain, infection, and hospitalization days. It also diminishes the effect of surgeon's hand tremors, as mentioned previously. The operative site is magnified into a three-dimensional image; there is a smaller incision, reducing blood loss, and the surgeon is comfortably seated at the console instead of standing at the side of the operating table. The cons are that the cost is higher, and somebody has to pay for it.

Many pose the question whether high-tech medicine is a misuse of resources or a miracle maker. Are Americans over treated? Some people argue that advanced technology is not actually improving health care. I disagree with this position. We know what health care was like in the 1960s and 1970s. There is no doubt that we are doing a much better job now, prolonging life and improving its quality, partly because of advanced technology and also because there's public awareness of its availability. The Katie Couric effect attests to that. Katie Couric, co-host on *The Today Show* at the time, became an advocate for colorectal cancer screening after losing her husband to cancer colon, prompting the public to demand colonoscopies. Couric underwent a colonoscopy on camera at the age of forty-three, which was not indicated, and explained each step of the procedure and its advantages. March of 2000 became the first national colorectal awareness month, and

colonoscopies have since become a well-known preventive procedure demanded by the public and approved by third-party payers.
The number of colonoscopy procedures has increased since then,
and the main issue now is how to use the awareness properly and
efficiently. The procedure is definitely indicated to reveal lesions
early enough to be completely eradicated and cured, but how frequently is it needed to be performed. Third party payers in combination with professional medical associations provide protocols
for implementation of procedures; the protocol for performing
colonoscopies yearly for sometime was changed according to the
patient's findings, condition and need, to every two, four or up to
ten year intervals.

I cannot wait to see how the Angelina Jolie effect will influence health care. Jolie, a well-known actress and humanitarian,
appeared in newspapers and on TV news, YouTube, and Twitter
when she revealed that she underwent a preventive double mas-
tectomy. Preventive surgery rather than curative surgery may be a
choice of the future; it is meant to be performed on high-risk individuals, who are presently possible to identify with the availability
of genomic and molecular testing. Angelina carried a mutation of
the BRCA1 gene, which increased her risk of developing breast or
ovarian cancer. (The BRCA1 gene is a normal tumor suppressing
gene that prevents uncontrollable cell growth, and therefore its
mutation might make it lose this function, lead to overgrowth of
cells and promote the development of cancer.) The mutation will
generally increase a person's risk from 12 percent to 60 percent.
Therefore, it is advisable for young ladies who have a family history of these cancers to have the screening test performed, and if
results are positive, may decide to undergo a preventive surgery.
A clear ethical protocol needs to be developed for the procedure
not to be misused. Treating cancer in the United States is already a $200 billion business each year. I wonder how this new

development will affect that cost, and I wonder how many beautiful young ladies will take these preventive measures.

There are many reasons, though, why technology might be overused; first, it reveals smaller lesions not identified otherwise, resulting in early detection treatment and an improved cure rate. Second, frequently the patient's complaint does not improve using simple diagnostic measures and treatments, necessitating further investigations, which require more advanced technology to get to the bottom of the problem. Third, doctors want to be sure they do not miss any hidden disease to prevent getting sued by the patient or the patient's family later for malpractice or negligence, so all advanced technical measures are taken. Fourth, patients know their rights and are aware of new technology because of advertisements, and they demand that everything be done, no matter how much it costs. They can do this because not a penny is coming out of their pockets; a third-party payer will pay for extensive investigative and diagnostic procedures, causing health-care costs to skyrocket. In addition, consumers do not see prices until after a service has been provided; even doctors do not know the cost of the procedure they are performing or the investigation they are ordering. Instead, payments are often the result of countless negotiations between a doctor, hospital, laboratory, pharmacy, and insurer, with the results depending on relative negotiating power. Each party wants to make a profit, no matter what it means for the patient. In fact, insurer's incentives to lower the cost are limited; they usually have the option to increase their premiums, as stated in fine print in their contracts.

More and more articles are being written about the cost of health care in the United States. The latest one I read in the *New York Times* was titled, "Paying Till It Hurts," and it tried to compare average prices in United States to other countries. They cited that an angiogram costs $914, versus $35 in Canada; a colonoscopy costs $1,185, compared with $655 in Switzerland; hip replacement costs $40,000, versus $7,731 in Spain; and an MRI costs an average of $1,121 versus $319 in the Netherlands. The United States spends 18 percent of its gross domestic product on health care, nearly twice as much as most other developed countries. Advanced treatment modalities with laparoscopy, endoscopy, and robotic surgery markedly improved health care and reduced hospitalization periods and time off work, but at what cost?

The staggering growth is taking place in pharmaceuticals also. Improved medicines with fewer side effects are constantly in the pipelines. The number of new medicines is enormous, yet the high price is really to pay for the amount of research and development that went into its production. The first step in creating medications is the discovery of a new compound, natural or synthetic, that affects a certain medical condition. This compound goes through several phases of experimentation to research its biological and chemical properties. Researchers determine: its effect on the disease as well as its side effects on nondiseased tissue and organs; how it is absorbed from the gastrointestinal tract if so administered and if anything prevents its absorption or is preferably given in a way other than orally; how it is distributed through the body and ultimately reaches the targeted organ; and how and when it is eliminated from the body, that is its "half life" so that the dosage and frequency of administration can be calculated correctly. They also make sure of its safety. Preliminary research is performed in the laboratory on tissue culture plates, and then on animals, followed by tests on healthy and sick volunteers.

The most accurate studies, as mentioned earlier in the book, are double-blind ones, using either the drug or a placebo (a fake pill). The doctor and patient are both prevented from knowing which of the two was administered. All this research is usually supported by the National Institute of Health; pharmaceutical

companies need to have the approval of the FDA and fulfill strict
regulations before they are issued the license to manufacture the
product. During this time, many compounds are tested and different doses are tried to develop the proper and effective drug.
It sometimes takes up to ten years to come up with the ultimate
prescription. Because of the extensive research involved, pharmaceutical companies patent their products, fix the price, and mo-
nopolize the market with their brands for several years before they
allow a generic replacement to be produced and flood the market
for a much lower price. Most drug patents carry the brand name
and are protected for up to seventeen years. The patent protects the
company that made the drug first and prevents anyone else from
manufacturing and selling the drug until the patent expires. Only
then are other companies allowed to manufacture the drug, and
the FDA must approve it as a generic replacement; it is then sold
at a much lower price, even though it has exactly the same active
ingredient. Only the color, flavor, and other inactive ingredients
might be different. Trademark laws in the United States do not
allow generic drugs to look exactly like the brand-name drugs.
Drug companies' frustrations with the FDA are slowly emerging;
there is a belief that the European Medical Agency is much more
thorough in its investigations, more transparent in enumerating
risk factors, and quicker in allowing the drug to be publicized for
usage. There is also a feeling that the FDA relies heavily on the
pharmaceutical and medical-device companies for its funding,
through charging user fees for reviewing drugs.

An article in the *New England Journal of Medicine* from January
2012 indicates that Lipitor was the top-selling prescription drug in
the United States in 2010, earning its manufacturer more than 7
billion dollars in total revenue, out of a twenty-billion-dollar market for high-blood-pressure medication. It has been estimated that
for statins, replacing the cholesterol-reducing brand-name drug

Lipitor, manufactured by Pfizer, with the generic equivalent in the year 2014, led to a projected savings of $4.5 billion annually. The use of statins when indicated and prescribed by a doctor is highly recommended, not only because it lowers the patient's cholesterol but also because it reduces the level of C-reactive protein, which is a sign of inflammation. In other words, statins help in reducing inflammatory processes in the body as a whole. More recently, the price of one share of the pharmaceutical company Gilead rose 2 percent in the stock market after the announcement that the FDA approved their drug Sovaldi and declared its use favorable for the treatment of hepatitis C, even in its late stages, and the price is going up progressively. The drug's sales exceeded those for any other drug, making a total of $2.3 billion in its first quarter on the market. Considering that there are three to four million Americans infected with the virus and many more millions in other countries and that the medication was proven to be highly effective if used in combination with Ribavirin, in addition to the fact that the treatment consists of one pill a day for twelve weeks only, the drug is highly recommended in spite of the cost. (One pill is worth a thousand dollars.) Each patient will cost the third-party payer an approximate $84,000 for a complete course of treatment. There are still some more drugs in the pipeline, the combination of which is being studied to combat the different types of hepatitis C. These medications would cost the patient, the government, or the third-party payer even more. Looking at it from the patient's and the general public's point of view, saving lives is worth that much. From the economical aspect, it is also worth it; this drug might be saving a lot of expenses that would have been incurred by treating the complications and progress of the disease without the help and curative results of such a prescription.

Popular over-the-counter medicines like cold medication, vitamins, anti-inflammatories, and digestive drugs are much less expensive; their cost is in the heavy uncontrolled usage without a doctor's prescription. It would be wise to reexamine the value of many health-related sacred cows that people indulge in just because of hearsay, such as antioxidants prevent cancer and heart disease, or vitamin D is good for you. I always want to ask, "Who said that?" It will help tremendously to dismantle some of the myths and misinformation so that people don't take a drug just because "they" said it is good for you. Statistics show that twenty-five billion dollars are spent yearly on dietary supplements and vitamins in the United States alone, even though vitamin deficiency has never proven to be a problem. As a treating doctor, I haven't seen a case of scurvy (vitamin C deficiency), beriberi (vitamin B deficiency), or rickets and osteomalacia (vitamin D deficiency) since I came to live in the United States. A big and costly industry exists to sell natural remedies, alternative medicine, acupuncture, herbs, and homeopathy; however, many of these substances are known to interfere with prescription drugs and are sometimes documented for being risky and costly remedies. I read an interesting book about this subject by Simon Singh and Edzard Ernst, *Trick or Treatment*. The authors evaluated alternative remedies and became convinced that there was a lack of scientific evidence of their effectiveness and that their dangers outweigh their benefits, which are mostly a placebo effect.

It always surprises me when I buy medication from the neighborhood pharmacy, and I am quoted a different price for a thirty-day, sixty-day, or ninety-day refill. The more I buy at a time, the lower the price per pill. Why do I pay $2 per pill if I take it for one month, $1.50 if I need it for two months, and $1 if I buy it for three months? If it were a candy bar, a banana, or a loaf of bread, I would pay the same price per unit whether I needed one, a dozen, or a month's supply, so what is the rationality in pricing medicine in this manner, other than the monopoly of the pharmaceutical companies? It is now a well-proven fact that people respond differently to medicines because different bodies react to drugs according to the individual's DNA composition. This is where, in the future, pharmacogenomics will replace pharmacokinetics in the standard of care and drug prescriptions. Instead of prescribing the same drug for the same disease or one standard dosage for everyone, treatment will be personalized. How much this will cost has not yet been studied.

Vaccination certainly has an unprecedented effect in preventive medicine; smallpox and polio have practically been eliminated, and childhood infectious diseases are very rarely encountered anymore. This reduces child mortality and leads to population growth. The flu vaccine is a lifesaver particularly for children, elderly, and immune deficient individuals, yet doctors and pharmacies provide them for all their clients on a yearly basis. Anybody who asks for the injection can get it, but at what cost? The vaccine needs to be reconstituted every year and produced de novo in view of the frequent flu virus mutation.

Physical therapy has tremendously good effects, and it eliminates pain in many unbearable situations. It assists people in regaining muscle strength after surgeries and improves muscle tone and joint movements, but it is often overused. Rehab, meaning "restore to normal," and physical therapy are popular and much indicated to the extent that kinesiology became a subject worth studying. This branch of science deals with the effect of forces upon the motion of matter, changing its physical and chemical system. It is approved by the American College of Sports and used for coaching players and dancers and treating their injuries as well as promoting general health and wellness. In the past, when someone complained that his or her neck had been hurting for some time when waking up, that person would have been advised to buy a new pillow or change sleeping positions. Today, things are different; one can simply make an appointment for physical therapy. Similarly, when somebody complains of back pain after prolonged sitting in front of a computer, he or she used to be told to place a pillow behind his or her back or to get up and stretch for a while. Now, that person needs to make an appointment with a physical therapist; similarly, when one complained of tingling sensation in the little finger after writing for a while, he or she would have been advised just not to lean on the elbow, for that puts pressure on the nerve reaching this finger and compresses it. Now, that person needs a full course of physical therapy and maybe ultrasonic treatment too, but at what cost? It does not matter; there is a third-party payer. It saddens me to see that even conscientious doctors take advantage of the third-party payer system. Some send reminders and e-mail their patients, advising them to do so. It is in the doctor's interest for the patient to visit before the end of the year rather than waiting till the appointment is necessary, just because the third party still has the money to pay. What a waste of the insurance company's money!

An architect I met who specialized in building hospitals said his firm was doing very well. They are continuously serving hospitals, adding new wings with more single-bed than double-bed patient rooms; remodeling emergency rooms, laboratories, and x-ray departments to fit the new machines and equipment and comply with new health regulations and environmental control; and providing for computers wherever needed. His company is also expanding the hospital cafeterias and family waiting rooms, sometimes equipping them with one or more TVs and children's play corners. Hospitals are competing like hotels these days to provide better care and comfort for their patients and to be labeled as five-star institutions, especially when local newspapers keep rating them for the public to compare, but at what cost? I enjoyed reading an article on this topic titled "The Good, The Bad and The

Ugly." It was about online physician reviews, and it outlined the pros and cons of using patient rankings to influence quality assessments and reimbursement for surgeons in an era of increasing access to electronic information. Google, Facebook, and various websites have become a profitable hospitality-and-service industry, offering information and reviews on practically everything. These websites assist the public in every aspect of life, including finding the best hotels and restaurants, quoting the best prices and routes for travel and booking vacations, and now there is increased traffic on physician- and health-care-centered websites. Patients find good, bad, or ugly information about doctors and health-care centers before visiting them, not even knowing the database from which the information was collected or on what factors the rating was based. In many cases, questions and answers were categorized as the following: overall rating, communication skills, bedside manner, availability, waiting-room accommodations, and friendliness of staff. None of these is really indicative of the doctors' ability to diagnose illness or cure a patient, and there is a great deal of concern about the authenticity of these reviews, so what are they all about—just another industry involved with health care, or a sales pitch? I could quote several questionnaires given to patients for comment after seeing their doctor. When the responses are tabulated, one can accordingly improve the facility. I would have found the information more meaningful if there were questions about how long the doctor spent with the patient; for example, did he answer all the questions you asked, and did you fully understand what your problem was and how it would be treated?

Unfortunately, the public does not appreciate doctors as invaluable healers like they used to; rather, doctors are marginalized and considered an avaricious group, part of an ever-growing high-cost health-care system. People forget that doctors are the backbone of the system. They are the ones who practice medicine and diagnose illness using the available tools. They counsel, prescribe medications, and perform the necessary procedures, using their education, knowledge, judgment, and skills. Their main problem is government and insurance company regulations, dictating what they can and cannot do by restricting or disallowing payments, yet doctors are required to use and blamed when not implementing every available diagnostic procedure and treatment measure.

Advertisement in health care is an issue of concern; it has never been deemed as illegal, but among physicians, it has always been considered unethical. Rules of ethics for the medical profession indicate that a physician, a group of physicians, or an organization (by advertisement) soliciting patients directly or indirectly is regarded as an act of self-advertisement and unethical conduct on the part of the physician. Advertisement is meant to be a marketing tool to persuade or manipulate a viewer and drive a customer toward a commercial offering and thereby generate increased consumption of a particular product or service and at the same time boost and promote the financial interest of the advertiser. Medical care has a different objective; it is meant to alleviate the sick from their pain and suffering, and medical practice is a humanitarian profession where self-exploitation finds no justification.

Advertisement could be traced back to the ancient Egyptians, who used papyrus as a medium; later, billboards became the main avenue for advertisement. Later still, radio broadcasters and newspapers took advantage of the growing business of advertisement. Presently, all forms of media have their share: television, digital and social media networks, Face book, twitter, LinkedIn, Google and other search engines are just some examples of entities that make money from advertisements, which became a several-million-dollar industry. It is estimated that medical advertisement accounts for 10 to 15 percent of the revenue of all traditional media,

TV in particular. Health-care marketing encompasses medical and surgical supplies, medical devices, information technology, innovative technology, pharmaceuticals, and drugs. The advertisement and promotion of medical products has been regulated and controlled since The Medicines Act of 1975 and its subsidiary legislation, The Medical Advertisement Regulation of 1977 (a declaration of the American Medical Association).

For a long time, companies hired marketing personnel and agents to drop by health-care providers' offices to promote and explain the effects of their new product in a scientific way, and the doctor would use his or her judgment regarding whether to use the new product. Since this became a profitable business, enjoyable TV shows are increasingly being interrupted by advertisements on health products and medicines to raise public awareness of what is new in the market. They advise viewers to ask their doctor about the drug in question and lead them to believe it's good for them; even though side effects and draw backs are mentioned the patient enters the doctor's office having already made up his or her mind not to leave without this particular new prescription. People listen to the advertisements and do not ask, "Is this medication really good for me, or is it simply going to be a profitable deal for the advertising company?" A consumer report indicates that 20 percent of patients request a prescription that they heard about on TV or through other means of advertisement. Viagra mania was so common that this drug was added to the admittance checklist in every ER. In other words, every male patient complaining of chest pain and rushed into the emergency room had to be asked, before the medical staff gave him any medication, whether he was taking Viagra!

To prevent the unnecessary use of advertised medications, a change to the regulation related to promoting OTC (over-the-counter) medicines has been proposed. The revision would be worded as follows: "Advertising for OTC is no longer allowed to be used in public media but only in professional media as medical journals." Another law that is a real breakthrough in terms of disclosure is the Physician Payments Sunshine Act, "which requires all drug and medical device companies to bare details of their financial relationships with doctors and teaching hospitals." This way, patients can decide whether the medication they were prescribed or the device they needed was profitable for the patient or for the doctor who prescribed it, recognizing that lawsuits have been filed against doctors mainly professors who were compensated by drug companies for promotional lectures, travel, meals, and related expenses.

It is saddening to see doctors and healers—who were known in the past to keep their phone numbers unlisted—now advertising like car dealers because of the competition. They make outrageous claims to being the best, the most advanced, the most talented, or the newest to solicit patients, rather than letting patients make their own choice and judge medical professionals according to their level of education, experience, reputation, skills, and bedside manner. There is a fine line between educating the public and exploiting them through advertising. It is clearly stated in the rule of ethics that soliciting of a patient directly by a physician or a group of physicians or an organization by advertisement or publicity through any mode so as to invite attention to his achievements is unethical. How do we reconcile the aforementioned ethical regulations against soliciting patients with the fact that an estimated $717 million was spent on hospital advertisement in one year? Since health care evolved into a medical enterprise, health-care organizations, HMOs, IPOs and PPOs are forced to compete for the consumer. In addition, because of the expanding cost of medical technology, the competition provides lower-cost medicines for the patient rather than better quality of care, while keeping financial gains for the insurer and for pharmaceutical and medical-device companies. This resulted in ethics of business overtaking the ethics of medicine. The Medicare program, which originated as a government plan to help the elderly is now relying on Medicare Advantage plans and the Health Insurance Marketplace, where insurance companies like Aetna, Humana, Blue Cross, Anthem, Cigna, AARP, Secure Horizon, and others are competing to sell Medicare patients their plans. They provide tables comparing coverage, out-of-pocket expenses, deductibles, drug availability, hospital affiliation, and service providers, leading to more confusion for the public. To find a health plan that fits your needs, you now have to go to a website or find an agent to guide you. Buying insurance to cover you and your family is similar to visiting a fairground, farmers market, or auction floor. It was so disturbing to open the Valpak envelope that I receive every week and find a 10 percent savings coupon for shoe repair, one for 30 percent off carpet cleaning, another for beauty salon products, and one promoting "eHealth that makes OBAMA CARE easy."

Patient advocates were heard, and to make sure patients get the best health care, the American Hospital Association provided a bill of rights in 1970, declaring that patients have the right to know what they could reasonably expect while in the hospital. In 2010, the Patient's Bill of Rights under the Affordable Care Act was designed to give patients protection in dealing with insurance companies, including the right to know about the extent of coverage, the amount of premiums, the choice of provider plans, the right to refuse a test or procedure, confidentiality, and the right to make complaints and appeals for new applicants. The Affordable Care Act also included a provision for Accountable Care Organizations (ACOs), where doctors form groups to collect data about the number of cases examined and protocols followed, the related efficiency, and the productivity risk factors and outcomes. All of these organizations measure quality, affordability, and accountability and then reveal the collected data to the public, presumably with integrity, in a transparent and ethical fashion.

At my age, when I get together with relatives and friends, we go for a walk, go shopping—rather, window shopping, visit a beauty salon, or go for a mild exercise; there isn't much more we can do. When we go to see a movie, many require glasses; others need hearing aids. When we meet for lunch, we choose restaurants that offer health food and that mention the number of calories in their dishes. We look for mostly natural or organic food, with no MSG or salt added. From the menu, we chose salads, veggies, and other dishes that contain good fats and good carbs and fiber, and we order little or no dessert. Our main subject of discussion involves what is healthy. We talk about the importance of exercise. Those who can manage it still go to the gym or fitness center, proud that they can afford to continue it; others are satisfied by a daily thirty or forty-five minute walk and recommend it, or they subscribe to Pilates or suggest curves, water aerobics or stretching exercises. Some of us watch every episode of *The Dr. Oz Show* and follow his advice; others listen to Dr. Sanjay Gupta and follow his recommendations. The most tech-savvy ones among us surf the net for answers to medical questions. The idea healthy diet is a mystery, because what really is healthy? All the diets I've heard described sound like food that tastes really bad and ruins one's appetite. One person said, "Stop eating white rice; brown rice is healthier." Another expert said, "Carbohydrates are fattening. Dark bread and whole-grain bread is preferable to white bread; it contains more fiber, which is healthy." This year, the fad is that all the previous diets were no good. We should be on a gluten-free diet, so go back to white rice, white bread, and less fiber. I personally do not engage much in these conversations; I know that what is healthy for one person might not be good for another. I prefer to quote what Mark Twain wrote about health (figure 23) .He said "The only way to keep your health is to eat what you don't want, drink what you don't like, and do what you'd druther not." Another quote is: "There are people who strictly deprive themselves of each and ever eatable, drinkable and smokable which has in any way acquired a shady reputation. They pay this price for health. And health is all they get for it. How strange it is. It is like paying out your whole fortune for a cow that has gone dry." One lady I know said, "I went to see my doctor for a checkup. Thank God everything turned out well, but he ordered a test I've never had done before to find out the level of vitamin D in my blood. It turned out to be lower than normal, so I had to increase the dosage of vitamin D supplements I am taking."

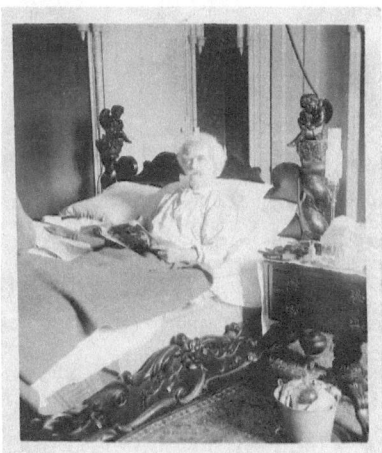

FIGURE 23

Another one said, "I changed my ENT doctor. It was strange: The new one told me I do not have any wax in my ears, but my old doctor used to tell me that I had a lot of wax buildup. He washed it out every time I saw him and charged me an arm and a leg for it."

A third one said, "My gastroenterologist advised me not to have my upper and lower endoscopies performed at the same time, but then I would be scheduled to have them performed on two separate days. I wanted to get done with them." Reimbursement for doing the procedures is different whether they are done separately or together. Conversations about doctors and medications often proceed similar to the following:

"I went to see my primary physician again. The antibiotic he prescribed previously did not work for me, so he put me on another one and told me that if it does not help, he will have to refer me to a specialist." "The specialist ordered a blood culture."

"I was shopping around for my medication. Can you believe it? The brand name ranges in cost from three to six times the price of the generic! I found it at Wal-Mart at half the price of my local pharmacy."

"I went for a refill for my blood-pressure medication; the price went up 10 percent, and my copayment also increased."

"Every time I eat out now, I get an upset stomach. I requested an ultrasound and CT scan from my doctor, he ordered them for me but found nothing; he sent me for an endoscopy procedure both upper and lower that was normal, and all the other lab tests showed no bad results. The doctor finally told me it might be stress." At what cost was this stress diagnosed? "My most recent lab tests showed high cholesterol, so my doctor called me to put me back on Lipitor, which I had stopped taking because of its side effects. After some discussion, he agreed to my not taking it if I followed a strict diet and exercise."

The medical community has been aware of vitamin D for centuries, but measuring the level of its metabolite, twenty-five hydroxyvitamin D, is the new fad that has become a subject of media advertisement in recent years. This hype, despite a lack of scientific evidence and data to back up its importance, caused every patient to request information about it, every general practitioner to order it, and every clinical laboratory to run the test. One reputable scientific study proved that vitamin D supplements did not reduce the progression of osteoarthritis. Another study linked high doses of the vitamin to an increase in bone fractures in the elderly, due to excessive brittleness of their bones. Whose recommendation should doctors and patients follow?

The other day, I accompanied a friend to the hospital. While I was waiting in the family waiting lounge for her to come out of surgery, I was surprised to be entertained by live music. It was one of the highest-rated hospitals in town. The public wants more and more, patients need better satisfaction, and families expect the impossible to be done, but when they receive the bill, they wonder why it costs so much. I would say that the costs come from industrialization, excessive advertising, and free enterprise.

HEALTH CARE, THE INDUSTRY

"I t's the economy, stupid," is a statement one hears frequently from people including businesspersons and entrepreneurs, especially when things go wrong or when the country is on the verge of a depression. During the Clinton campaign, these same words uttered by him, helped the governor of Arkansas become our president; sure enough, his administration markedly improved the economy in the United States and around the world. The national economy is the complicated system that comprises production, distribution or trade, and consumption of goods and services, and it involves a series of transactions. Economic activity is connected to natural resources, minerals, oil, precious metals, and agriculture as well as creativity, education, productivity, and the formation of corporations and organizations that assist with labor and employment; it is accentuated by an acceleration process, reduction of costs, and opening new markets, with diversification and supply meeting demand.

Adam Smith (1723–1790) was considered the first true economist during the Age of Enlightenment and industrialization. His general contribution to society was his inquiry into the nature and causes of national wealth. He did not believe the accepted theory that it depended only on a nation's natural resources. In his breakthrough book, *The Wealth of Nations*, published in 1776, he was critical of government regulations, and he argued that the reason for success was self-interest. His book also addressed a better use of labor and the forces of supply and demand as well as the advantage of competitive business and the implementation of laissez-faire to assist the economy. He described an invisible hand, a concept wherein each individual is being led by an invisible force toward self-good. Today, automation, advanced technology, and information technology add a great deal to the national and international economic growth. They have raised productivity, improved the quality of goods and services, and reduced labor hours. Economic growth goes hand in hand with industrialization and the production of goods and services. In particular, it depends primarily on extracting resources (raw materials), secondarily on sending them to factories (manufacturing), and thirdly on services needed, such as management, financial, intellectual, marketing, and operational. These relationships culminate into the formation of businesses, companies, and corporations responsible for production or involved with trade, usually privately owned or with some government assistance, to create a profit at each of the many steps involved. This economic system, referred to as capitalism or free enterprise, is intended to provide for the general population and simultaneously increase the wealth of the owners. There are several organizations in the United States that monitor the economy very carefully; some are governmental, and others are privately owned. These include the National Bureau of Economic Research, the Bureau of Labor Statistics, the Bureau of Economic Analysis, and the Census Bureau. They set up the following economic indicators to monitor economic growth closely: the manufacturing index, jobless claims, consumer satisfaction, vendor performance, manufacturers' new orders, building permits, money supply, interest rate spread, and the consumer expectation index. These factors apply to health care the way it is provided now. Therefore, it is definitely an industry, privately owned, with government assistance for the poor and elderly; it affects and is affected by the national economy, and its cost depends on the extraction of raw material (drugs), manufacturing (equipment and machinery), and services rendered, and thus it requires not only doctors and medical professionals but also: financing, management, forming of corporations, rebuilding hospitals, and human resources, accentuated by the modernization of supply and excessive patient demand.

Doctors used to open more than one office in different districts of town to accommodate their patients, but because they are now reimbursed less for their services, they share offices. This is evidence that you are dealing with a competitive market. You hear about laboratories that run blood tests merging into one large facility and big drug manufacturers advertising that they conglomerated into one, or you see small hospitals on the verge of bankruptcy, closing their emergency rooms or trauma centers because they cannot afford to care for indigent uninsured patients, and they are ultimately taken over by big corporations. When this happens, you can be sure you are dealing with an industry, with all its business-related mergers and acquisitions. You are no longer dealing with the art of healing as medicine used to be considered. Marsha Mercer, a freelance journalist, recently wrote an AARP article titled "Merger Mania." She wrote about hospital consolidation, explaining that it was good for hospital business but not so beneficial for patients. She claims that CEOs of small hospitals, to stay afloat, find themselves under severe pressure to cut costs and are therefore obligated to form partnerships with doctor's practices and other health-care providers or merge and affiliate with larger institutions, resulting in an increased cost for their patients (larger institutions usually charge more because they give more advanced services). More than a hundred hospital deals took place in the year 2012, and it is expected that one thousand hospitals in the United States will have new ownership in the next seven years. Compare this analysis to the old days. In the year 1873, there were only 178 hospitals with a total of 35,064 beds in the entire Unites States. In the year 1909, the number of hospitals increased to 4,359, with 421,065 beds available. By 20 years later, the number of hospitals grew to 6,665, with a total of 907,133 beds. The majority started as community hospitals, built and managed by donors and churches that served as boards of directors, but now they are managed by big corporations.

This distinction between business and private enterprise prompts me to mention a personal experience. Lately, because of the economic depression, rising unemployment, and fading economy, I have been getting more and more phone calls from companies advertising their businesses. I hear the ring, answer, the phone, and listen to a recording that says, "We will be in your neighborhood next week, and we can pass by to introduce you to our cleaning product—" Before they finish the sentence, I hang up, uninterested. I have also received advertisements for cleaning air ducts and maintaining my refrigerator or vacuum cleaner. Junk mail has doubled in volume. One letter I opened read, "You have been chosen for a free estimate of our open-door bath tub, especially fit for the elderly." I am a senior citizen, but I am not ready to get involved in any remodeling now, so it went to the trash. I don't usually care much about advertising, but one telephone call really turned me off. It was a recorded message that said, "One of our physicians will be in your area, giving a talk about a new drug for respiratory problems. If you are elderly and have problems with breathing, please call us back at [the provided phone number] to make a reservation." There was also a letter that interested me enormously, from a hospital to which I like to donate every once in a while. The letter included a very intelligently worded pamphlet about a privately owned company that works with that particular hospital, Life Line Screening; in the letter they emphasized the importance of the power of prevention for people with no prior symptoms or warning signs of certain conditions. In essence, the letter raises public awareness that the blood tests usually ordered by doctors for a yearly checkup are not enough to identify your risk or predisposition to a serious illness, because they may not show certain hidden diseases. This company offers screening tests that doctors do not routinely order because insurance companies and Medicare do not pay for them unless the patient already complains of symptoms that would require and allow for these tests, and that might be too late for some individuals. The company claims that they have already screened eight million men and women and saved thousands of lives. They also mentioned that they will be in my neighborhood for one day only and asked the community to register in advance because of the limited number of appointments they can take. They offer five tests for just sixty dollars each, and surprise, surprise: They also have a sales pitch. They offer all five tests together for a special price of $149, with a savings of $120. Is that what medicine, the art of healing, has become: an enterprise offering a sale?

As I mentioned before, when I needed medical care in 1958, I paid a reasonable fee for a limited service; that was the system. You paid out of your pocket for your health care. If you had the money, you could seek the best care, and if you didn't, you would only be provided minimal care or none at all, or you would be a burden on the government that would provide help for free. In 1964, I needed similar medical attention in Germany, and I did not pay one dime out of my pocket. I now know why the German system was set up that way. It all started when Otto von Bismarck, a conservative German statesman, instituted antisocialist laws. He introduced several insurance programs, including health insurance. As far back as the 1880s, Bismarck had a general antisocialist agenda, but he felt that a little bit of socialism might prevent it from becoming full blown. Bismarck also cared about the German workers and therefore invented the welfare state as part of the unification of Germany in the nineteenth century. He introduced the first health-insurance system that was later implemented similarly in France, Belgium, Switzerland, and the Netherlands. The system started with the poor then included all the rest of population. It started with health and grew to include accident and disability. The three key principles were: (solidarity, government responsibility and subsidierity.) The system used an insurance plan in which insurers have what was referred to as "sickness funds," financed jointly by employers and employees through payroll deductions. The plan was required to cover everybody and not make a profit, and doctors and hospitals were private. Things started to change at the time of the Weimar Republic, (1919) when the socially minded cooperated with government to implement reform with new policies that included providing health care to citizens and noncitizens alike. It was also during this period of time that the focus of health care shifted from private and individual patient health to preventive medicine for everybody. The Bismarck system of care is implemented in Germany to this day.

There are also other systems of health care that exist. The well-known Beveridge model, named after the social reformer William Beveridge, was designed for the British National Health Service. In this system, health care is provided and financed by the government through tax payments, most hospitals and clinics are government owned, and doctors are government employees. Health care is therefore free for everybody using this system; no one pays a penny out of pocket. This tends to be a low-cost system, because the government controls what doctors can do and what they can charge. There are, in addition, some private hospitals and specialists that can give more advanced services and charge their patients for them. This model is also applied in Spain and most of Scandinavia. The Canadian health system is a mixture of the two previous ones I've described: Health providers are from the private sector, but payment comes from a governmental insurance program that has no financial motive and into which every citizen pays. Therefore, it is a national health-insurance program that is well regulated and simple to administer, and its costs are controlled. However, the problems with the system are that patients frequently have to wait longer to be seen and treated, and the medical services that can be provided are limited. If a patient requires more than what the system provides, the payment has to come out of his or her pocket.

After living for one year in Germany and admiring their health-care system, my husband and I were granted another fellowship in the United States for the year 1964–1965. We felt that we had entered a new world, and many things were different; it was the country we used to hear about, the land of freedom, opportunity, and human rights. Even though in Germany, hospitals were clean and well organized, we were stunned by the elegance of the private hospitals in the United States. They were very well equipped, clean, advanced, and up to date. Corridor walls were decorated with fashionable paintings, and some hospital rooms looked like rooms in five-star hotels. Patient beds were motorized and on wheels, chairs in the rooms were on wheels, and there was a TV for each patient to watch as desired. But it was shocking to see how different all that was from the government hospital, caring for the poor and needy, less than one mile's distance away. It was obvious that the system of fee for service worked well for the haves, while the have-nots were not so lucky. Equal rights to health had not yet been granted.

Just before we left at the end of our fellowship in 1965, the general public and the news media hailed President Johnson, who was courageous enough to sign the Medicare Bill. The bill was passed to legislate that the government would assist citizens over the age of sixty-five who had retired, lost their medical coverage from work, and found it impossible to afford or be provided coverage by private-insurance companies. The bill also covered the disabled and those with renal failure; the system was based on the model of private insurance, which was fee for service. The Medicare bill was signed into law on July 30, 1965, in Independence, Missouri, at the Truman Memorial Library. At the ceremony, the president paid tribute to former president Harry Truman, who attended the event. In 1945, Harry Truman had a vision of how a government program can positively affect a change in social environment. He had asked Congress for legislation to establish a national health insurance plan but could not get it done. In other words, former president Truman was honored in 1965 because he was the first chief executive to endorse health insurance under social security 20 years earlier, but failed.

The idea of considering government health coverage actually started in the United States when the influential AALL (American Association of Labor Legislation) publicized the need for workman's compensation in 1906, an effort that culminated in thirty states passing such a law in 1915. However, a subsequent proposal for a general national health insurance failed at the time of Woodrow Wilson, who won the presidential election of 1912. National health insurance was opposed by the life insurance companies, whose business was directly threatened, and physicians were unwilling to submit to any management by federal or state government. The administration and funding of health insurance was not considered to be the government's role. Earlier in US history, the founding father Thomas Jefferson was also wary of government power; he felt that the country would best prosper by remaining a nation of individualism. His views of laissez-fair dominated, and the idea of freedom for private enterprise prevailed within the medical industry. One of Jefferson's famous sayings was, "The government is best which governs least." This philosophy, combined with the philosophy of social Darwinism (i.e., survival of the fittest) kept the government from interfering in ameliorating people's hardships. Instead, its role was to stay out of their business and push for a natural evolution of society; therefore, Congress defeated any government attempts to be responsible for health insurance. The most forceful opponents were the insurance companies led by Frederick L. Hoffman and the Pharmaceutical Manufacturers' Association.

The pharmaceutical industry tops the list of the most profitable industries in the United States, with a 17 percent return on revenue. National expenditure on pharmaceuticals today accounts for approximately 30 percent of total health-care costs, in spite of the availability of generic drugs competing with brand names. The pharmaceutical industry in fact began in Europe with the scientific revolution in the seventeenth century and soon spread with the Industrial Revolution and its increased productivity. For example, Merck started as a simple pharmacy, originating in Germany in 1668, and it industrialized in 1827 as a company in drug manufacturing all over the world. Bayer AG was founded in 1863; it was extremely famous for its production of aspirin in 1899, and it became part of a well-known German chemical company conglomerate that manufactured dyes, I.G. Farben. It is now one of the biggest pharmaceutical industries. It has an interesting history: A businessman, Friedrich Bayer and a dyer Johan Friedrich Weskoff were friends, because of curiosity they worked in their kitchen and discovered how to make a dye "Fuchsine."They founded their first start up and sold dyes derived from coal-tar to the textile industry. From 1881-1914 the company grew into a big industrial research company that included pharmaceuticals, and in 1899 its chemist Felix Hoffman launched Aspirin into the market. He produced it to help his father who suffered from arthritis. The company's growth was interrupted during the war, lost most of its assets including its US patent and trademark that were confiscated. Where there is a will there is a way, and after losing in two wars "Bayer is still one of the largest industries."Similarly GlaxoSmithKline originated in 1715 and did not become industrialized until the nineteenth century. Pfizer was founded in 1849 in the United States by two German immigrants aiming for a better life in the land of freedom and opportunity, and ended up being a huge industrial complex

In the year 1920, the CCMC (Committee on the Costs of Medical Care) conducted the first national comprehensive study of medical economics and issued several recommendations for changing the medical practice; they recognized that health care had become unaffordable for many families and individuals. It took several years of study to investigate and research potential economic solutions and to propose an organizational design. Finally, they came up with a recommendation in 1927, suggesting that medical services should be provided by physician groups, costs should be distributed over persons and time using an insurance program, funds and services dedicated to disease prevention should be increased, and community agencies to coordinate medical-care services should exist. Yet their recommendations did not include compulsory government health insurance, and the ideas were mainly rejected by the AMA (American Medical Association). The private-insurance model was still the most favorable approach. The nation prided itself on freedom and private enterprise, and the economy was doing well, so why make any changes? Unfortunately the country later plunged into a deep economic collapse, the worst recession ever. In 1933, millions of Americans found themselves out of work, and unemployment became a huge problem. The philosophy of the general public and President Franklin D. Roosevelt changed. They believed that it was the government's duty to care for its victimized citizens, and several agencies were established to combat the depression, including the drafting of the Social Security Act in 1935. Congress passed the act, which provided benefits to retirees and the unemployed as well as assistance to the states from the federal government for implementation. The act included (Titles 1,111,1V, V, VI and X).The government announced a plan to consider affordable health care at this time. Unfortunately, this again drew immediate protests, and a sickness-insurance plan was abandoned; the excuse was that the quality of medical care might be affected. The present state Medicaid programs to care for the health of the poor were only created in 1965, the same year Medicare was enacted by the Social Security Amendments. It added title XIX to the Social Security Act as an entitlement program from the government to assist states in providing medical coverage for low-income families and individuals. This was during the same year my husband and I were busily making the best out of our stay in the United States, working in research and finishing our publications before getting ready to go back home. We felt young and healthy, so we did not worry about our own health care, and therefore were not very excited or concerned about the changes that were implemented. We personally had no coverage at all, and we were lucky we did not fall sick during our stay; it would have cost us an arm and a leg. We went back home, to our fee-for-service system and out-of-pocket payments.

We later came back to the United States in late 1969, this time to stay, so we needed to live the American way. We were bombarded by sales people knocking our door: including the encyclopedia Britannica and shelves that carry them, vacuum cleaner and the Avon lady. We bought a car, and it had to be covered by car insurance; we bought a house, and it had to be covered by home insurance. And one of our friends introduced us to a nice man who was an insurance agent; he worked for a big company that offers life and health insurance and explained the system in detail. Health care in United States differed from what we had experienced before, at home or in Germany or Britain. This agent said that he needed to sell us life insurance to assist the family after our death and health insurance to keep us alive and to provide help in paying the medical bills when we get sick. "Otherwise, you might lose your shirt and everything you own," he said. "If you are not insured," he said, "some doctors may not be willing to treat you, and hospitals might not even admit you, except for an emergency. That was really scary, so we sat and listened to his advice. I discovered later, when I worked as a doctor, that what he had said was very true. If you do not carry an insurance card in your wallet, you are labeled a cash patient, and cash patients are not usually welcomed unless they have an emergency condition. Who would pay their bill? I also noticed that when one visits a doctor's office, after the receptionist warmly greets you, that person would ask for your insurance information before inquiring about your health needs. While practicing in a hospital, I personally witnessed a circumstance like the one this agent mentioned. A semi comatose man, probably in his early sixties, was admitted to the hospital through the emergency room. He was reported to be a cash patient, so the hospital administrator and his primary physician decided to transfer him to the county hospital as soon as he gained consciousness and was therefore fit to be transferred. Otherwise, he would cost the hospital a fortune. When he did regain consciousness and was able to talk, it was discovered that he was a rich businessman who was not medically insured because he felt that paying the insurance premiums was a waste. He was generally in good health and could afford to pay his bill in case of sickness. Therefore, he was not transferred to the county medical center and was locally properly treated. When my husband and I learned how health insurance works, the agent explained the following details: the differences between insurance companies, what their limitations were, how the premiums were calculated—depending on age, gender, and risk factors and the outcome of your physical exam and blood test results—how the premiums could be lowered if the deductible was raised, how preexisting conditions affected the rates or might be excluded from coverage, how some employers provided their employees with medical insurance, and how the system works for the self-employed. We enrolled and paid our premiums for years, but luckily we were young and healthy and did not cost the company a penny for a long, time. However, our premiums grew each year, according to the inflation rate and our increasing ages. It was not a coincidence that when I drove through town, I started noticing the names of these insurance companies appearing on more high-rise buildings and thought, "Wow, they must be making a lot of money."

Private medical care and doctors' compensation for services was not a concept first implemented in the United States. In fact, it goes as far back as the 1780s BCE, practiced in Mesopotamia (between the rivers Tigris and Euphrates), the land that saw many civilizations, including the Sumerians and Babylonians. Campbell Thomson and Franz Kocher published history previously only available on cuneiform and clay tablets. In Mesopotamia, under the section of the Code of Hammurabi titled "in sickness and in health," it was expected that if a physician, particularly a surgeon, was successful in helping the patient, that doctor was to be paid more. A failed surgery cost the surgeon more, meaning that compensation and liability were to be determined by the patient and his or her family.

In the United States, the concept of fee for service changed over time, and the first of what could be called individual health-insurance plans became available during the Civil War. The plans were first restricted to accident insurance that provided coverage for injuries related to accidents or travel. Later, Massachusetts health insurance offered group policies with a comprehensive list of benefits in 1847. Later still, disability insurance was provided; lastly, sickness insurance. One of the major health-insurance companies in the United States at present is Blue Cross. It was developed in 1929 to cover teacher's hospital care, and it then extended to other employee groups. Blue Shield, the second-largest, developed by employers in lumber and mining to provide medical-care payments for physicians, and was founded in 1939. Both remained the largest companies insuring most private patients. In 1982, they both merged into one company, Anthem, "too big to fail."

During President Reagan's administration in the 1980s, drastic changes occurred in legislation that affected business. The TEFRA law was one of them, changing tax brackets and reducing them markedly for the higher income class and eliminating several deductions that raised taxes paid by the middle class. The second law, the one that affected health care, was the implementation of the DRG (diagnosis-related group) system, which created a new way to reimburse hospitals for their services. The law was intended to replace the cost-based system that was used beforehand, where each service rendered was paid for separately. The DRG would classify hospital cases into one of 467 groups that identified the product that a hospital provides in anticipation of its use for reimbursement; the system was implemented in1982. It determined how much Medicare should pay the hospital as a lump sum for each "product," based on the disease, diagnosis, procedures performed (if any), patient's age, sex, and outcome on discharge, rather than paying for each patient as an individual for the care that person received, like charges for hospital bed, lab tests performed, surgical suite and medication. Each so-called product had a certain code number, and a code book was established. The ICD (International Statistical Classification of Diseases) and the

CPT (Current Procedural Terminology) were meant to standard-ize classifications of claims for billing purposes, ignoring what was actually done for each individual patient and ignoring the diagnostic procedures, time, and effort the professional put into each case. Doctors were also compensated for their professional work accordingly and had to use the code system in their billing. Insurance companies realized that this system would lower hos-pital and doctor payments and applied it too, and no doctor could bill for his job as a health care provider unless he or she used the same ICD code numbers used for billing for the care provided. That was a drastic change in the way a hospital, doctors, or any health provider was reimbursed. No wonder entrepreneurs took advantage of the situation and consulting firms gave birth to a new industry of providing fee-maximizing advisor seminars. Hospitals and doctors found an incentive in using coding specialists to make sure they were not under-coding and therefore underpaid.

Before the DRG system was implemented, most people who were privately insured and not yet eligible for Medicare were covered by something referred to as indemnity insurance plans; they would pay the health-care provider a big percentage of the fees, amounting to 80 percent, and the patient would pay the re-maining part other than the agreed-upon deductible. The higher the deductible, the lower the premium, and the patient was free to choose his or her doctor, but when the cost of health care skyrocketed, cost containment became the name of the game, the health-care system had to be reformed, and managed care started to develop. This involved the formation of HMOs (health maintenance organizations), PPOs (preferred provider organiza-tions), and IPAs (independent practice organizations), and doctors rushed to be part of them. They did not want to be left out and lose their patients to the organizations whose aim was to charge less and pay less and thus lower the cost. Most doctors wanted to be part of this new system, but some kept their private practice and their patients.

HMOs are large organizations that can buy medical services for thousands of people and make a decision about what type of care those individuals will receive and therefore, they can lower health-care costs for individuals and employers. Patients joining HMOs pay low premiums but can only see doctors, use providers, and visit hospitals that belong to the network. These doctors and providers agree by contracts to treat patients in accordance with the HMO guidelines and restrictions and accept lower fees for their services in exchange for a steady stream of customers. Patients who sign up with an HMO are also required to choose one of the organization's primary care physicians (a gatekeeper), who will be in charge and who has to get approval from the HMO to continue the patient's care, including referrals to a specialist and sending for x-rays, lab tests, and special procedures or hospitalization. All of these referral facilities must have special contracts with the HMO and accept the reduced payments for their services. The HMO pays a flat fee for the medical services rendered, agreed upon by the original contract, resulting in cost control; it also gives an incentive for a restrictive practice. For example, if a general surgeon whose main practice consists of hernias, hemorrhoids, and gallbladders is paid a fee for the service of performing a surgery, he or she would be inclined to do it. But if the doctor is paid a monthly flat fee for seeing a hundred patients per month, why would that surgeon perform the procedure unless it is absolutely necessary or the patient is in real danger if the surgery is not immediately done; that is cost containment as applied by HMOs.

The Ross-Loos Medical Group, established in 1929, was considered the first HMO in the United States, "though this term was not used at that time." It provided services to the department of water and power employees, and when it started, enrollment was at a cost of $1.50 per person per month; later, the fire department, the police department, and the telephone company (AT&T) joined. They restricted themselves to outpatient clinics and used private hospitals for their inpatients; it wasn't till the early 1970s that they built their own hospital. I worked for them for one year, was not very comfortable with their system, and quit. During my stay, I had the chance to watch Dr. Ross himself, still operating with relatively steady hands at the age of ninety. He was famous for operating on parotid gland tumors. Donald Ross and Clifford Loos were two originally Canadian doctors who pioneered what was called at the time "the prepaid group practice." Patients and families had to register for membership and pay a monthly or yearly premium, and then they were examined and treated for free. The term HMO came into being only in the 1980s, but it applied the same system. These organizations hire their physicians as employees, using what they call a staff model. It's a captive group that is not allowed to see any private patients. Alternatively, the organization may contract with groups of doctors (IPAs, or independent practice associates) as is the case with Kaiser Permanente, a more recently developed HMO in California.

The rush to form other types of health organizations started in late 1970s and early 1980s with the PPO mania that also led to the formation of EPOs (exclusive provider organizations). Similar to the HMOs, in the PPOs, (preferred provider organizations), participating providers also belong to a managed-care system of doctors, hospitals, and other health-care providers who covenanted with an insurance company or third-party administrator to provide health-care services at reduced rates to insurers' or administrators' clients (but not as low as the HMOs), and negotiate with them to a set fee schedule. Patients can see any of their contracted doctors, choose any hospital they prefer, and are not restricted by a gatekeeper. So, insurance companies that used to pay health providers a fee for service now pay according to the organizational agreement, whether it is an HMO, EPA, or PPO, and the procedure that they pay for has to be allowable and authorized by a reviewer according to the contract. Likewise, they pay hospitals a certain amount according to the DRG rather than what service was rendered, saving quite a lot of money for the insurance company. It is obvious that a member of a PPO pays a higher Insurance premium than a member of an HMO.

In spite of all these organizational changes and all the attempts to lower the cost of health care, and although doctors accepted reducing fees and hospitals lowered charges, the cost of medical care is still on the rise. I think the secret is that all these managed-care organizations, HMOs, EPOs, PPOs, and even Medicare, still have their contractual agreements with the same third-party payers, including Anthem, Humana, Aetna and United Health, the same insurance companies, and their business is to make money. One can enroll with any one of them as a member of an HMO, EPO, or PPO. The administrative costs and CEO salaries of these private-insurance companies and the formation of all these organizations are rising; advances in science, technology, and expensive machinery keeps enabling more and more diagnostic and curative procedures. Patients are living longer, and families are demanding that more be done.

With the implementation of Obama Care, medical-insurance companies were compelled to provide more services and provide more coverage—for example, for preexisting conditions, that will cost them more, so they raised premiums on their members or canceled their insurance policies. Hospitals and doctors will be reimbursed less for their services to their patients and will have to bear the brunt of admitting or seeing a greater number of patients. There will be stricter regulations for patient hospital stays and readmission, and the number of low-pay Medicaid patients will increase. Health providers will suffer and are in the process of rethinking and rearranging their priorities, regulations, and business models. Some hospitals are already closing departments and reducing their services; others are closing their free clinics, and competition for hospitals to improve their image to look like five-star hotels is diminishing. Doctors are applying for membership to hospitals that are for profit, rather than the Medicare-approved ones. They are also refusing to take Medicare and Medicaid patients, telling their old patients that they will accept them only if they pay cash. A new specialty is resurfacing, the concept of the concierge doctor, whom the patient can have an agreement with to be taken care of for a yearly retaining fee, exactly like he or she can retain a lawyer to call for advice twenty-four-seven rather than making a trip to the doctor's office.

Doctors are rethinking how much industrialization of health care took place and how far technology interfered with patient care. One hears them reiterate that patients are out of touch; diagnostic tools replaced patient examination by auscultation, palpation, and percussion. Robots replaced surgeons in performing surgical operations, and extensive specialization led to patients who had to see several doctors to get each of their organs treated separately. This model has replaced the previously individualized doctor-patient relationship. Another way of thinking is in the process of adopting what is referred to as "socialized medicine"—that is, health care using social media. There are already several privately owned health-information technology companies that own electronic health records and provide health-care information directly to the public, such as Dr. Jay Parkinson, Hello Health, MDVIP, and Medical Encyclopedia. Sick people can surf the net, post their complaint, find their reports, diagnose their illness, and perhaps learn about treatment without worrying about the patient privacy act. And then they can make an educated guess about whether they want to see their doctor and prepare to discuss how they want to be treated. All these innovations show that there is definitely an urgent need to establish an equitable system for health-care reform as well as for providing and paying for medical services.

THE CODE OF ETHICS

S ince the inception of the art of healing, there has been awareness of the ethics and morals involved during the practice of
medicine. The Hippocratic Oath that physicians used to abide by
and follow very conscientiously was for a long time the only code
dealing with the relationship between the medical caregiver and
the people he or she cares for, including teachers, students, and
peers. There were add-ons to the code of ethics over the years, and
changes were made depending on patients' needs and practices.

With the onset of religious beliefs, Jewish thinkers and Roman
Catholic scholars contributed a lot of moral and traditional issues.
However, the first book dedicated to medical ethics, *The Conduct
of a Physician*, (Adab el Tabib) was written by a Muslim thinker,
Ishaq Ibn Ali al-Rahawi, who lived in El Sham, present-day Syria,
during the eleventh century. He considered the physician a guard-
ian of the soul and body and wrote twenty chapters on topics
related to medical ethics. He was referred to as Hakeem, meaning
"wise man," but also used for doctors. He wrote about *hisbah*,
referring to quality assurance, licensing, record keeping, practice
standards, and malpractice.

In recent decades, many changes that happened in the medical field can be attributed to wars and their effects, including
war crimes and misery, depression associated with poverty and
famine, and other economic concerns as well as extensive regulations and reforms and a higher level of responsibilities lay
on the shoulders of medical professionals. The code of ethics
needed to be amended to keep up with events. One example of

a change (or addition) to the code of ethics is the Declaration of Geneva, which was adopted by the World Medical Association in 1948 after war atrocities were realized. It added a declaration of physicians' dedication to humanitarian goals; it was amended in 1968, 1984, 2005, and 2006 in accordance with new developments in the health system. The original wording of the Declaration of Geneva was as follows:

> *I solemnly pledge to consecrate my life to the service of humanity*
> *I will give to my teachers the respect and gratitude which is their due;*
> *I will practice my profession with conscience and dignity;*
> *The health and life of my patient will be my first consideration;*
> *I will respect the secrets which are confined in me;*
> *I will maintain by all means in my power, the honor and the noble tradition of the medical profession;*
> *My colleagues will be my brothers*
> *I will not permit consideration of religion, nationality, race, party politics or social standing to intervene between me and my patient;*
> *I will maintain the utmost respect for human life, from the time of its conception, even under threat;*
> *I will not use my medical knowledge contrary to the laws of humanity;*
> *I make these promises solemnly, freely and upon my honor.*

Eventually, the phrase stating that everyone has the right to live from conception to death was removed. Did that change the ethics of medical practice, or was the change needed because of changes in the law of the land?

Health care has always been an integral part of the multiple activities of many departments of the WHO (World Health Organization), and the American Medical Association adopted the first code of ethics in the United States in 1847. It concentrated on four main issues. The first was autonomy, meaning the patient has the full right to choose or refuse any treatment. The second was protection, meaning one should act in the best interest of the patient. The third was do not harm, which is self-explanatory. The fourth was justice, and that included fairness and equality in distribution of health resources and in the decision of who gets what; it had not been established or achieved till our present time. Later, because of the expansion of the medical field, the NCEHC (National Center for Ethics in Health Care) was founded in 1991. It provided analyses and guidance on controversial ethics issues affecting not only the patients but also health-care providers, managers, and makers of health policies. Its main office is located in the central office of the Veterans Administration in Washington, DC, and its staff includes law makers, educators, theologians, and social workers, among others.

Ethics has always been an issue of concern in medicine, but it is becoming more and more so since the art of healing has become a complex field and a business that integrates science and advanced technology with the art of compassion. In fact, some question if the term "health care" is now a misnomer and argue that the new terminology should be "the medical industry." It has never been so critical to bring an ethical prospective of compassion, respect, and justice to these spectacular diagnostic and curative procedures to ensure that patient care is delivered wisely and well. Therefore, ethics has an extra significant role in health care, particularly considering that several industries have a high stake in it, and multiple issues need to be considered as part of the code of ethics. Needless to say, the most important issue is still regarding the morally right and wrong and appropriate and inappropriate actions as well as maintaining integrity to the highest degree; there are also legal responsibilities to be aware of, relevant business issues, and fraudulent and deceptive behaviors. Health care is no longer a one-to-one patient-doctor relationship but more of an organizational one, and therefore there are more privacy and confidentiality issues than in the past.

Because there is a lot of advertisement for new drugs and medications as well as the use of advanced technology and instrumentation, the Internet, and other forms of information technology, there are numerous vendor-doctor relationships, and there may be some conflicts of interest. DTC (direct-to-consumer) advertising and the promotion of medicines, devices, and screening tests are legally allowed only in New Zealand and the United States and only since 1997. Because of the advent of unusual interventional procedures, the patient's informed consent and its wording and delivery to the patient are of utmost importance. According to an article in the bulletin of the American College of Surgeons from August 2013, the term "informed consent" first appeared in a malpractice case of *Martin Salgo v. Leland Stanford Jr. University Board of Trustees* in 1957. The plaintiff alleged that he was not informed about all the risks of a procedure he underwent under anesthesia, and he ended up with a complication. The ruling in favor of the plaintiff stated that sufficient disclosure of risks and complications (informed consent) was necessary for patients to make appropriate autonomous decisions. Patients are now not only told verbally about the risks but also have to sign a written consent form that enumerates all risks involved, even the possibility of death. Many times this scares the patient and makes him or her nervous, uncomfortable and think twice before entering the surgical suite.

The first legal decision addressing this issue in the United States took place in 1914. A judge in the New York Court of Appeals ruled that a surgeon was guilty of battery because of his decision to remove a tumor he found in a patient's abdomen while performing another abdominal surgical procedure and not telling her beforehand. In this case, it was obvious that the patient's right to autonomous decision making was her defense. The ruling of Justice Cardozo's in this case was, "Every human being of adult years and sound mind has the right to determine what shall be done with his own body and a surgeon who performs an operation without his patient's consent commits an assault for which he is liable." There is a lot of debate now about two issues of ethical concern that need to be resolved: Is abortion an issue of doing no harm or one concerned with autonomy? The other issue is about patients treated in university teaching hospitals: Are they consenting to residents in training or fellows being present in the operating room assisting, finishing up the procedure, or doing minor procedures; and if the patients are not consenting, are they aware of the role of these residents who are still in training? Many times, patients wonder about doctors they are not familiar with making rounds and examining them.

"Are they, residents, fellows, or associates," a patient might ask.

A third ethical issue was the topic of discussion during a session on surgical ethics at the 2014 Clinical Congress of the American College of Surgeons. The discussion centered on the informed consent the patient signs before the operation and the content of disclosure, including benefits and risks. The surgery is meant to improve the patient's health, which is identified as physical, mental, and social well-being. Therefore, is it advisable to include the cost and financial impact, for example, the extra cost for robotic surgery, regardless of the patient's insurance status or only in case the extra cost must come out of pocket? The patient's well-being after surgery should include absence of disease with no financial side effects.

Discussions about mandates are nowhere to be found, probably because they contradict the fundamental principal of autonomy. However, as medical professionals are ultimately the ones who see the effects of public policies on health care and its costs, some health organizations like the American Board of Internal Medicine and the American Society of Internal Medicine decided that they need to play a role in public decisions related to health care and public safety. They cited as an example the overturn of the helmet legislation of bike riders and motorcycle drivers. The doctors take care of these patients when they end up in emergency rooms with severe trauma deleterious to their well-being, no matter whether they are covered by insurance or they will be a burden on the taxpayer. They concluded that doctors should have a say on such legislations. Their opinion should be heard.

In the mid-1980s hospitals tried to improve the health-care system and competed in implementing the idea of having trauma centers to increase readiness in treating cases with severe injuries secondary to involvement in accidents. Emergency rooms expanded, surgeons and anesthesiologists who were on call slept in their hospitals to assure immediate availability, since early interference is of utmost importance. New equipment and emergency supplies were provided, and many lives were saved. Unfortunately, many trauma patients proved to be indigenous and uninsured, and they became a burden on the hospital budget. Participating hospitals were on the verge of being financially ruined, so one by one, big hospitals opted out of the program and closed their trauma centers. Now the question is whether a mandate of a provision that improves health care and public safety infringes on an ethical or philosophical right of autonomy. The right to act autonomously finds support in both US law and in basic principles of Western biological ethics, and it is manifest in Justice Cardozo's statement from the aforementioned case. But the judge did not comment on the quality of the individual's decision, whether good or bad, what risk he was willing to take, or how this decision would affect other people's rights or interfere with general public health. Therefore, mandates need to be a subject of serious discussion.

Because the medical business and industry became so diversified with the involvement of gigantic insurance companies, HMOs, hospital associations, pharmaceutical companies, information technology, and federal and state government, how are these entities making combined decisions for protecting the patients' interests? It takes a lot of cooperative decision making to protect the industry interests and at the same time, not hurt the patient's interests and protect his or her rights. Many organizations are involved, many rules and regulations are put on paper to be followed, and the wording of ethics in medicine keeps changing accordingly year after year. The Federal Trade Commission and US Department of Justice police the hospital mergers, and many states also require mergers to be approved by the state attorney general to assure adequate hospital availability, sometimes blocking a hospital consolidation that might hurt the community. The FDA is in full control of the safety of medications and prescriptions, but many of the pills in vogue that are said to contain necessary vitamins, minerals, and herbs are not under its supervision. HCFA (the Health Care Financial Administration) was established in 1977. Its rulings state the final opinion, clarification, and interpretation of complex laws related to Medicare and Medicaid utilization and peer review. A division of the Centers for Medicare and Medicaid Services, an agency and department of the Health and Human Resources, administers Medicare and the federal part of Medicaid, and it oversees health financing and establishes standards for medical providers that require compliance to meet certain requirements. It oversees enrolling beneficiaries and processing premium payments.

Another regulator watching over properly provided health care is the (JCAHO)Joint Commission on Accreditation of Health Care Organizations (now TJC, The Joint Commission), a private nonprofit organization that initially started as the Joint Commission on Accreditation of Hospitals (JCAH) in 1951; it used to inspect hospitals to identify problems, if any, and assure good patient care. In 1965, when the Social Security Act was established, it accredited hospitals not only for licensing but also to make sure they met all Medicare conditions before they could accept patients covered by Medicare. Policies and procedures were reviewed, departments and books inspected, quality of care and safety measures revised. A hospital has to pass the inspection, or given time to correct the citations, if not accredited after that it is not allowed to accept Medicare patients. Because the medical field had expanded, in 1987, JCAHO expanded the scope of its activity, and its mission changed to focus on continuously improving the safety and quality of care provided to the public by providing support and improved services and care. It is now governed by a twenty-eight member board of commissioners, including physicians, nurses, medical directors, administrators of health insurance and other health care, consumers, providers, employers, labor representatives, health-plan leaders, quality experts, educators, members of the American College of Surgeons and the American Medical Association, and last but not least, ethicists. Together, they put forth the rules and regulations for how medicine should be practiced in the United States. It is definitely not a simple art of healing anymore.

In spite of all these governmental and private agents, knowing how best to deal with health care and how to reform it is still a dilemma. Health care is unaffordable, the cost is rising, and not everybody is covered; one has to strike a balance between improving the quality of care and cutting costs. Everybody agrees that any health-care system has to be sustainable in the long run and that every member of society must have adequate accessibility to health care. However, there is argument about the contents and limits of coverage, and there continue to be discussions about the clarification of responsibilities and accountabilities of stakeholders. What are the ethics of equitability, setting limits, rationing, the absence of code requirements, and setting up advanced directives, living wills, and powers of attorneys? Procedures that were never heard of in the past require a lot of education for doctors, nurses, and the public. How does a doctor feel when he or she writes a note on the patient's chart, and the order says "Do not resuscitate"? And what does the respiratory therapist think about the instances wherein he or she is called to perform CPR and, in the process, breaks the patient's ribs or, managing the ventilator as a final resort in vain, and then is finally given instructions to turn off the machine and disconnect all the wires to let the patient go and rest in peace? In what conscience does this person face the family and explain what is happening when some family members understand and expect this decision to be made, and others still beg the doctor do everything possible to save the patient's life, even if it is only for a few more weeks.

End-of-life choices are extremely difficult to decide upon for both doctors and patients and their families. Therefore, the ethics of having advanced directives and living wills are often stressed. It should ultimately be the patient's decision to indicate what his or her desire is. It is easy to find fault with both doctor and patient and with the patient's family. Someone might accuse doctors who use a fee-for-service model, doing everything possible to save their patients no matter how pointless it is, of excessive treatment to make more money. On the other hand, some HMOs are accused for not doing enough for their patients, just to save money, and they are blamed for possible homicide. More commonly, doctors are fearful of litigation and do whatever they are asked with little feedback to avoid getting in trouble. Many patients are reasonable enough, and when a procedure is suggested, they would comment that if it will lead them to have a better quality of life, so be it. I heard some patients say, "If I am not going to be me anymore or have any kind of quality of life, then let me go."

Others said, "If I come down with a terminal illness, I wouldn't want to spend my last months or the money that I could leave to my family on futile care." Comfort care is always desired, but prolonging pain and suffering feels inhumane; therefore, the help and support of hospice is many times advisable. There, the terminally ill who are more realistic about their condition are given help to alleviate pain and suffering. They receive comfort and palliative treatments to live and die in dignity, with no active interference or futile measures, and this gives them better final days. Amazingly, some studies have found that people placed in hospice care often live a little longer than patients who have the same disease and seek active cures.

"Futility" is a term used more and more among medical professionals, and therefore it needs an ethical consideration. The phrase "medical futility" refers to interventions that are unlikely to produce any significant benefit for the patient. It concerns both qualitative benefits of the intervention—that is, improvement of quality—and quantitative benefits, where the likelihood that an intervention will benefit the patient is exceedingly poor. Since the goal of medicine is to help the sick and improve the patient's life, the doctor has no ethical obligation to offer treatments or procedures that do not benefit the patient. Futile interventions that would only increase pain and suffering in the final days are ill advised, even though a patient's autonomy allows him or her to ask for it. Now the problem arises regarding who decides when a particular treatment is futile. Ethically, futility determinations should conform to more general professional standards of care, not decided by each individual doctor at the bedside, unless the patient because of his or her autonomy decides against a particular intervention. On the contrary, the patient's family may insist for the procedure to be performed even though the health-care team considers this particular intervention to be futile. The rationale for the decision to withhold the procedure needs to be passionately explained in such circumstances. By contrast, an experimental treatment might be considered and suggested, with full disclosure that empirical evidence of its effect is lacking and still unknown. The biggest issue that needs to be emphasized is that futility does not mean rationing, and the intervention is refrained from because there is a lack of its benefit not because of its cost. If this is explained, patients and their families can often embrace the idea and feel comfortable with it.

Euthanasia another term that is questionable and should not be confused with futility, originated from the Greek word, "good death" it started to be debated a lot when doctor Kevorkian, a pathologist nick named as "Doctor death" declared that he was a euthanasia activist. It was alleged that with his assistance, he allowed and advised patients in misery how to kill themselves, and this was considered assisted suicide. The first apparent use of this term was to describe how the Emperor Augustus (63 BCE–14 CE), the first emperor of the Roman Empire, died without suffering in the arms of his beloved wife Livia, the rumor was that she had poisoned him. Painless inducement of a quick death is felt by some to be more compassionate and humane than a prolonged painful miserable end stage of life, yet euthanasia is still illegal in most developed countries, and religions do not allow it because it entails one person intentionally killing another, even though there is no personal gain in doing so. Others consider it mercifully permitting a person to have his or her wish to be relieved from prolonged pain and suffering, this being one of the person's ethical rights (autonomy). Doesn't the patient have the right to die as well as the right to live? There is an argument that voluntary euthanasia should be permitted if the patient consents to it because he or she has the ethical right for autonomy in decision making, in contrast to involuntary euthanasia, where there is no previous patient consent. Again, during major depressions, individualistic conservatism that praised "laissez-fair economics" and its followers encouraged the movement for euthanasia. (It solves the problem of the excessive cost and rising health-care expenditure incurred by the terminally ill.) Euthanasia became lawful in Belgium in 2002, the third country to legalize it after Luxemburg and the Netherlands.

On a health-care blog, I came across an article about how doctors die. It's not a frequent topic of discussion, but doctors die too. They know enough about medicine, the science involved, and the technology available, but they know its limitations too. What's unusual is not how much treatment they get compared to most Americans but how little they want to be done. They have seen and done every effort to save their patients, but also sometimes wonder why families let their loved ones to get cut open, perforated with tubes, hooked up to machines and assaulted with drugs at the end of their lives, its futile. They sure have their reasons, they want their loved ones to be treated get the best care and everything possible done to live a meaningful life. Doctors don't realize that their own families feel the same way and want everything to be done for them; they do not feel it's futile.

Cost containment and cutting services in health care is a

major concern for people writing rules and regulations for utilization and quality-assurance reviewers. The ethics involved,
particularly that cost containment is already being slowly implemented in many ways in big institutions and among big corporations, emphasize that the changes do not negatively affect the
consumer—that is, they are eliminating waste, not cutting needed
services. An article in an issue of the journal of the College of
American Pathologists talks about a united front against waste by
controlling test utilization, claiming that one of their procedures,
after eleven weeks of implementation, reduced the charges for
daily phlebotomy, blood drawing, from $147.73 to $108.11. This
was done simply by announcing each week to the house staff
and attending physicians the dollar value that had been charged,
assuming that realizing how much it costs would raise awareness
and make the ordering doctor think twice. They also developed
more precise normal ranges for tests performed, thereby limiting
erroneous abnormal results and thus eliminating the unnecessary follow-ups and further investigations of false positives.
Another procedure that is still in the evolutionary stage is for
the pathologist, not the treating physician, to be in control of test
ordering. The article noted that in the United States, the treating
doctor orders as many tests as he or she desires for his patient to
find out what the patient has and what the problem is, whereas in
the United Kingdom, the doctor requests tests to be formulated
by the laboratory, according to the disease diagnosed, so the pathologist would assume the responsibility of saying something
like the following: Doctor, tell me what's wrong with your patient,
and we in the lab will decide, based on the clinical presentation,
what tests are to be provided. This saved a lot of waste. I do not
believe this difference in the way of ordering lab test is a matter
of saving and lowering the cost. I believe the reason goes deeper
than that. In the United Kingdom, health care is not for profit. In

the United States, medicine is an industry with the value of laissez-fair, and therefore it will be considered a conflict of interest if it is left for the laboratory director to order the laboratory tests. It is a matter of business ethics. Grouping tests into tiers is another possibility not yet implemented. Tier 1 would include tests that any general or primary care physician should have open access to, while tier 2, which tend to be more expensive, would only be available to specialists; and tier 3 tests would only be offered to expert panels. The reasoning is that there are so many new tests on the market right now, some that haven't even been proven to be accurate, sensitive, useful, or necessary; many times patients hear about these tests from advertisements or chats with friends and request for them to be ordered by their doctors, and the doctors agree. Pathologists came up with these ideas for lower costs in laboratory testing. Similar provisions need to be recommended and applied to other expensive diagnostic procedures such as CT scans and MRIs.

Other cost-cutting measures that are already in place involve having the specialist examine the patient and make the diagnosis and important decisions in the line of treatment, and then having a PA (physician assistant) or NP (nurse practitioner) take care of follow-ups, answer patients' phone calls, and give some limited advice. The PA or NP, being paid less than the doctor, saves the third-party payer and lowers their cost, but how ethical is it, and how much does it save the consumer? The availability of procedures needing expensive technology, whether diagnostic or curative, such as open MRI or robotics, could be limited to use only in special hospitals or tertiary centers. It may also be useful to clarify the indications and favorability of preferring the use of an expensive robot to a general surgeon's laparoscopic procedure.

Hospital utilization committees always recommend early patient discharge to lower unnecessary charges, and they assume that prolonged stay might make patients more prone to nosocomial (hospital acquired) infections. Keeping the patient one or two extra days in the hospital till he or she fully regains strength might be less costly and also more ethical than having the patient readmitted after early discharge due to unexpected complications. Present Medicare regulations disallow paying for early readmissions during a certain period of time after discharge, thus saving money for the government, but this is a loss for the care providers, and the expenses come out of the taxpayer's money. Another option is to form transitional care groups of doctors who would follow up on discharged patients to prevent or take care of complications when they occur, so as to prevent readmission, and this is less costly.

Some think that the growing trend of doctor's specialization needs to take a step back, and specialists need to regroup and cooperate more to gather all of a given patient's information together and to treat each patient as a whole, not each organ separately. Bundling patient information may be the new trend, and software engineers should be working diligently to provide a collecting system. The days of privacy are behind us, and social networking is the game of the day. Everybody posts details of his or her private life on Face book or Twitter, and one can perform an Internet search on any name and get all available information. It is unethical to declare patient information because there is a privacy code, and yet it would be more practical and less costly for the doctor to get all the information he or she needs from a central database or an electronic device rather than each doctor carrying a laptop or tablet around with the required information. The United States is one of the slowest countries to adopt HIT (health information technology) for fear of encroaching on the patient privacy act; it ranked eighth after other developed countries that have a fully integrated hospital and clinic system, such as Great Britain and Germany. We are trying to implement it now, after the Obama administration came up with HITECH, the Health Information Technology for Economic and Clinical Health Act as an economic stimulus bill in 2009 to encourage the use of IT in the health industry. Under this act, the Department of Health and Human Services spends millions of dollars to promote and expand the adoption of health information technology and to create a nationwide network of electronic health records as a foundation for health reform.

Many businesses are now using EDW, enterprise data warehouses, which are a unified database that holds all business information and makes it accessible across the company and to other interested industries. This was found to be a powerful management system. Since health care is now a multidisciplinary business, services for electronic medical records have been founded that could support retrospective and population-based analysis in the form of a technological interface containing well-integrated, clean, and formatted clinical, administrative, and historic patient data. An example is the Regional Medical Laboratory that, with its enterprise data warehouse, now contains data on more than two million patients, going back as far as fifteen years. The system is worth the massive amount of money pouring into its development and usage. It offers a high level of security, and its data mining is enabling professionals to make decisions that can influence cost and revenue, optimize patient care, resource utilization of preventive care, predict drug susceptibility and microbiological resistance, and many more aspects of follow-up in health care, in a relatively ethical way and considering patients' privacy.

Since health care changed from being an art of healing to a medical enterprise, lowering costs and making it equally available for everybody has been an ethical dilemma. No measures taken have been very effective until now, and we did not reach our goal. The problem is how the volume of patients treated can be increased, combined with lowering the cost, without sacrificing the quality of care. The brunt of cost containment is mostly directed toward the consumer, the patient, and the health-care providers. How about the other side of the coin? The industry could start with raw material that is less expensive, lowering the cost of manufacturing drugs—maybe outsourcing with good quality control—and the production of technological tools; they could find sources of money for research and development other than taxpayers' money. How about getting lawyers out of the malpractice deals and encouraging settlements in cases of true malpractice and convincing medical insurance companies and their shareholders and CEOs that enough is enough? Last but not least is concentrating more on preventive medical care.

There are genuine cracks in every health-care system. Under the Affordable Care Act, insurance companies still have a say, affecting its affordability, as insurance companies are for-profit businesses. In the British National Health System, the government does not have the means to give the best expensive care, which may cause a long wait for patients and a delay in services. Similarly, in the Canadian system, there is a cap on what services are provided. We need a treatment balancing act that prevents the tradeoff between individual and population health and a careful balance between resource allocation and cost containment. We also need a middle point between a revenue-driven health-care system that incentivizes high costs and focusing on population-level health care that incentivizes underuse and lower costs. This approach must also try to get the patient, who became out of touch because of the extensive use of high tech, back in touch by more frequent use of palpation, auscultation, and percussion.

It is ultimately up to the general population to make the difficult choice and decide how they wish their health to be treated and managed. With so many changes over the years and the effect of science, technology, automation, IT, and innovations, the art of healing, which was based on consciousness, religious beliefs, and ethics, turned into a medical enterprise; and with new codes of ethics related to business and affected by the country's economy, the primary code of ethics also changed from simply abiding by the Hippocratic oath to abiding by its amendments and the many rules and regulations emphasizing corporate and business needs and legal issues. In an effort to reduce cost, autonomy, the first item in the code of ethics, has been lost to regulations from Medicare, PPOs, and HMOs. Protect and do not harm, the second and third codes, gave way to laissez-fair, no code, directives, and powers of attorney interfering with decision making. Privacy and confidentiality issues of patient's rights disappeared with the introduction of IT, social networking, and computerization. Advanced technology procedures, both diagnostic and curative, with a high cost on the third-party payers, rendered it impossible to implement the fourth code, justice and fair and equal distribution of health-care resources.

So, before trying to fix our broken health-care system and implementing changes, members of the public need to be educated about the pros and cons of each choice they make. Cutting costs is a valid option, but where, how, and for who remains an ethical question. Pouring more money into research and development is another valid option, improving the general population's health and reducing sick days; this, in turn, reduces unemployment and disability and improves the economy, rendering health care affordable for everybody.

Soon, medicine will go through the biggest shake-up in history from the implementation of the science of individuality. We will have mobile medicine. We started using mobile phones more than three centuries ago. The first one was sold for four thousand dollars, designed only to be used in the car and to function only in certain areas of coverage in the vicinity of the widely spread cell towers. The prototype weighed 1.1 kilograms and was 23 centimeters long, 13 centimeters deep and 4.45 centimeters wide. The battery used to be placed in the trunk and the handset in front, and one had to go through an operator to place a call. With improvements over the years, it became a handheld gadget every person, child, adult or elder carries around and uses all day. In addition to calling relatives and friends, the smart phone is used for e-mailing, broadcasting, reading books or news, advertising, social networking, and connectivity with the world; one can surf the net and search for any information needed. It replaced watches, for it tells you the time; it replaced the camera, for it takes pictures for you with improved resolution year after year. Pathologists like me took advantage of this function and, by using a small adaptor and developing a new iPhone app known as Pocket Pathologist, they can attach the smart phone to a microscope, take pictures of the slides they are examining, and share their views with fellow pathologists on the spot for consultation and better diagnosis. The mobile phone replaced maps, for it can give you directions and even inform you of traffic problems. There is no more need for dictionaries; the phone can help you with that and do all the translations for you, and it serves as your flashlight in the dark. Now with the age of digital technology, we will be able to digitalize human beings like was done before with sound and light. Nanosensors can be embedded and relay information from the body to smart phones via wireless networks, similar to but more sophisticated than the wrist watches that can read your pulse, blood pressure, and sleep phases. The smart phone will change medical care from being shaped by rules, regulations, and guidelines scaled to the population at large, to individual patient monitoring and individualized treatment. The smart phone may soon prescribe diagnostic apps and be able to read your EKG and echogram.

Digital technology will assist in each patient using his or her genome at a biological, physiological, and granular level to determine appropriate preventive and therapeutic measures. There is a trend toward more laboratories with the ability to perform an individual's genome-wide scans. There is also a tendency for more and more people to be interested in knowing about their genetic predisposition and their risk for diseases, so as to take preventive measures and seek early treatment. However, there is an ethical controversy: Should the testing be left to the choice of the public, or should it only be performed by doctor's orders? Another consideration is whether knowing the risk factor is going to affect the person psychologically and how this information will be kept private so it does not affect the person's life or job or get used in a discriminative or exploitative fashion against the patient, either in daily life or in a malpractice suit. A new set of codes of ethics other than GINA, the Genetic Information Nondiscrimination Act (2008) needs to be developed before genomic testing is publicized.

In a previous chapter, I mentioned my granddaughter telling me that she could not wait to see how technology is going to change in the next ten years. I can now tell her that at least in the medical field and health care, it will definitely change markedly toward the better. With all the advances in biomedical sciences, health information technology, digitization, and wireless electronics, the routine molecular digitization of humankind is just around the corner. We will need to deal with the continuous changes happening inside our bodies and outside effects on them, and therefore will have a health-care database called Wikinomics similar to Face book and LinkedIn, another one, microbiomics for all species of bacteria that live inside us, like in our mouths and gastro intestinal tract, metabolomics for our end products of metabolism, epigenomics for environmental conditions affecting us, genomics for genetic sequencing, and proteomics for splicing of our proteins. The new techniques necessitated a new medical vocabulary to be used with the application of -omics, a field of study in biology since this field has become such an increasingly data-rich subject. The suffix -omics is added onto previously used biological terms to allow the addition of more and more data for novel insight. Futuristic possibilities are surely tremendous. We will see amazing advancements, and we will experience individualized affordable medical care for everybody to live healthfully and happily ever after, with a brand new code of ethics.

To summarize, we went back to ancient times, through the age of science and enlightment, age of technology, age of industry and now all that is left to say is:

Welcome to the digital age.

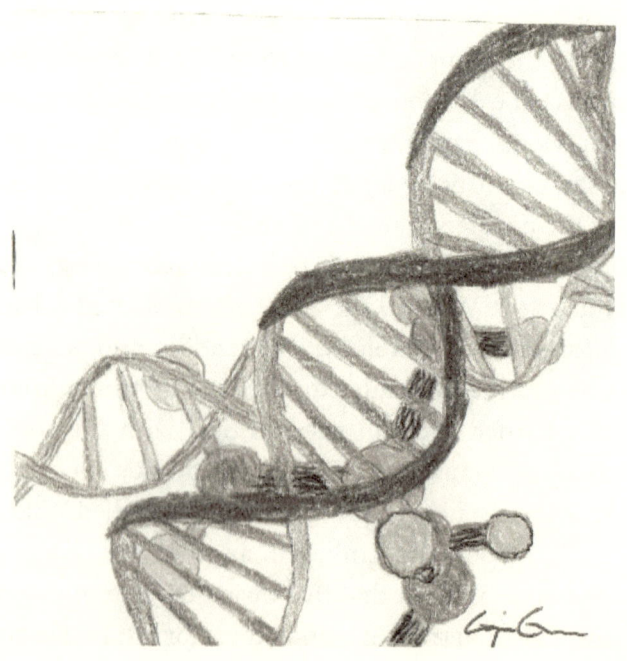

ILLUSTRATIONS

Figure 1: Heidelberg University. Courtesy of, Universitat HIEDELBERG, Kommunikation und Marketing, Internetredaktion.Bildredaktion, Grabengasse 1,69117, Heidelberg.

Figure 2: Schistosoma life cycle. Courtesy of [CDC] Centers for Disease Control and Prevention USA Government.

Figure 3: Hippocratic Oath, from the historical collection. Courtesy of the US National Library of Medicine. USA Government. Bethesda MD.

Figure 4: Ebers Papyrus [1550 BC] Courtesy of the [NLM], National Library of Medicine USA Government Bethesda MD.

Figure 5: Edwin Smith papyrus [1600 BC]. Historical collection courtesy of [NLM].

Figure 6: Healers, [NLM] historical collection.

Figure 7: Hippocratic Oath, from the historical collection, US National Library of Medicine.

Figure 8: Materia Medica. From the Dioscorides Codex Spain 12th-13th centuries, courtesy the Bernard Becker medical Library, Washington University School of Medicine. Saint Louis MO.

Figure 9: Plant in Materia Medica from the Vienna Dioscorides Codex, courtesy the Bernard Becker medical library.

Figure10: Eye of Horus talisman. Attribute to: Anthony Rudd, at Robert Harding Picture Library, Nicholson House, Berkshire,SL6 1LD.

Figure 11: Church and School of Wicca. Courtesy Yvonne and Gavin Frost founders.

Figure 12: Pentagram. Courtesy Yvonne and Gavin Frost.

Figure 13: Khamsa. Courtesy Ali Akyus at the evel eye jewelry store

Figure 14: Horus Stamp. Courtesy the Ophthalmic heritage and Museum of Vision, The foundation of the American Academy of Ophthalmology.

Figure 15: Gray's anatomy, from the medical book club of sciencebookaday, 1858, American Wellcome Library, and courtesy Amanda Smith, the body sphere ABC radio National.

Figure 16: Digitalis Purpuera. Attribute to Glen Kopp. Information Manager Missouri Botanical Gardens.

Figure 17: Aspirin Logo, Courtesy of Bayer Intellectual property, Gmbh,Global Trademark Center.

Figure 18: Bayer building, New Jersey, USA . Bayer Intellectual property, GmbH, Global Trademark Center.

Figure 19: Salix Alba Willow Tree, Attribute to Bruce Marlin, Red Plant Inc.

Figure 20: Male catkin, Attribute and thanks to Marcel Zurreck. Oberdorfstrasse 11,8808 Pfaffikon, Swittzerland

Figure 21: Dr, Debakey, and Courtesy of Gwen Pitman at NASA media services.

Figure 22: Genome.DNA credited to the US department of energy Genomic science Program.

Figure 23: Mark Twain credited to: Barbara Schmidt, independent researcher, writer and consultant.